PANCREATITIS
DIET GUIDE
And
COOKBOOK
For the Newly diagnosed

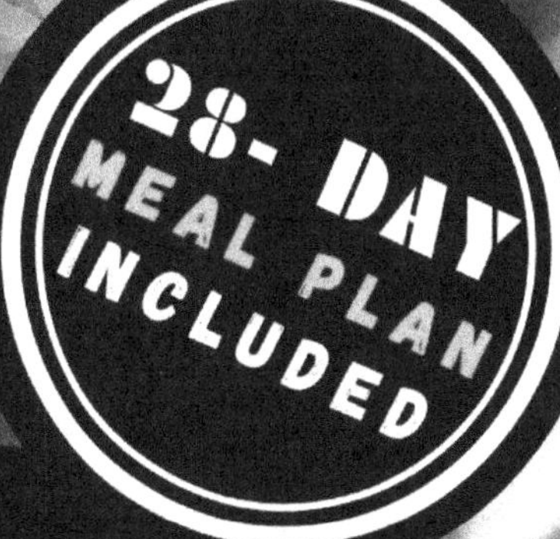

SAY BYE TO
ABDOMINAL PAIN,
VOMITING, NAUSEA,
RAPID HEART RATE,
LOW BLOOD PRESSURE AND MANY OTHER SYMPTOMS
YOU MIGHT BE EXPERIENCING.

(2 in 1)
PANCREATITIS DIET
GUIDE
and
COOKBOOK
For the Newly Diagnosed

Wholesome Low-Fat Recipes to reduce inflammation and Kiss Pancreatitis Symptoms Goodbye – No More Abdominal Pain, Vomiting, or Fatigue plus 4 weeks meal plan to reverse pancreatitis

Judy Kelly

Table of Contents

Introduction

Dear readers,

Embarking on a journey toward better health often begins with a profound moment of realization. A diagnosis of pancreatitis, whether for yourself or a loved one, is undoubtedly one such moment. It marks a turning point, a juncture where lifestyle choices take center stage in the pursuit of well-being. Welcome to "Pancreatitis Diet Guide and Cookbook for the Newly Diagnosed." This comprehensive guide is not just a collection of recipes; it's a roadmap to navigating the challenges, embracing a specialized diet, and rediscovering the joy of food in the face of pancreatitis.

Understanding Pancreatitis:
Before we dive into the culinary realm, let's first unravel the complexities of pancreatitis. In the opening chapters, we aim to demystify the condition, exploring its various types, symptoms, and the diagnostic journey. Understanding pancreatitis is a crucial step toward informed decision-making and empowers you with the knowledge needed to embark on a path of wellness.

Importance of a Specialized Diet:
Pancreatitis demands attention to dietary choices like few other conditions. In this cookbook, we emphasize the pivotal role that a specialized diet plays in managing symptoms and promoting overall well-being. From the science behind the choices to practical tips on incorporating pancreatitis-friendly ingredients into your meals, we aim to guide you toward a healthier relationship with food.

How This Cookbook Can Help:
This cookbook is your companion, designed to simplify the complexities of adopting a specialized diet. It goes beyond recipes, offering practical insights into essential kitchen tools, pantry staples, and fresh ingredients that will elevate your cooking experience. Each chapter is a step-by-step guide, from breakfast options to satisfying snacks and hearty main courses, ensuring that flavor and nutrition coexist harmoniously.

Consider this book not only a source of culinary inspiration but also a holistic resource for your well-being. We delve into essential aspects of managing pancreatitis, including tips for dining out, stress management techniques, incorporating physical activity, and building a support system.

Embracing the Culinary Journey:
Cooking with pancreatitis may initially feel like a challenge, but we encourage you to see it as an opportunity for culinary exploration. Our recipes prioritize both health and flavor, proving that nourishing your body can be a delightful and fulfilling experience. Let this cookbook be your ally as you embark on a journey toward better health, savoring the flavors of a pancreatitis-friendly lifestyle.

Together, let's turn this moment of diagnosis into a catalyst for positive change, embracing not just the joy of cooking but the joy of living well with pancreatitis. Welcome to a new chapter in your culinary and wellness journey.

Sincerely,

Judy Kelly.

Chapter 1: Navigating the Pancreatitis Diagnosis

A. What is Pancreatitis?

- Pancreatitis, a term derived from the inflammation of the pancreas, is a medical condition that demands attention and understanding. The pancreas, a crucial organ located behind the stomach, plays a pivotal role in digestion and blood sugar regulation. When the pancreas becomes inflamed, it disrupts its normal functioning, leading to a cascade of symptoms and potential complications.

Pancreatitis can be acute or chronic. Acute pancreatitis is a sudden inflammation that may resolve with proper medical intervention, while chronic pancreatitis involves persistent inflammation that can lead to long-term damage. Understanding the nature of pancreatitis is crucial, as it sets the stage for informed decision-making regarding treatment and lifestyle adjustments.

B. Types of Pancreatitis

Pancreatitis manifests in different forms, each presenting its unique challenges and considerations:

1. Acute Pancreatitis:
    - Occurs suddenly and is often linked to gallstones or excessive alcohol consumption.
    - Symptoms may include severe abdominal pain, nausea, vomiting, and fever.
    - With prompt medical care, acute pancreatitis can often be managed, and the pancreas can recover.

2. Chronic Pancreatitis:
    - Develops gradually over time, often due to long-term alcohol abuse or other underlying conditions.
    - Symptoms may include persistent abdominal pain, weight loss, and malabsorption of nutrients.

- Management focuses on pain relief, addressing nutritional deficiencies, and preventing complications.

Understanding the specific type of pancreatitis is crucial for tailoring treatment plans and lifestyle modifications to the individual's needs.

C. Symptoms and Diagnosis

Recognizing the symptoms of pancreatitis is essential for early intervention. Common symptoms include:

1. Abdominal Pain:
   - Often starts as a dull ache and may progress to severe, persistent pain.
   - Typically located in the upper abdomen and may radiate to the back.

2. Nausea and Vomiting:
   - Accompanies abdominal pain and may be triggered by eating.

3. Fever and Rapid Heart Rate:
   - Signs of inflammation and potential infection.

4. Changes in Bowel Movements:
   - Diarrhea or oily, foul-smelling stools may indicate malabsorption.

5. Unexplained Weight Loss:
   - A consequence of malnutrition due to impaired pancreatic function.

Diagnosing pancreatitis involves a combination of medical history, physical examination, and diagnostic tests. Blood tests, imaging studies (such as CT scans or MRIs), and sometimes endoscopic procedures are utilized to confirm the diagnosis and determine the severity of the condition.

D. Emotional and Lifestyle Impact

A diagnosis of pancreatitis extends beyond the physical realm, profoundly impacting emotional well-being and lifestyle. The chronic nature of the condition, in particular, may necessitate a reevaluation of daily routines and habits. Emotional responses can range from shock and disbelief to anxiety and depression.

1. Emotional Impact:
   - Coping with the uncertainty of chronic illness can be emotionally challenging.
   - Feelings of frustration, fear, and sadness are not uncommon.
   - Seeking support from healthcare professionals, support groups, or mental health services can provide valuable resources.

2. Lifestyle Impact:
   - Dietary adjustments become a cornerstone of managing pancreatitis.
   - Limiting or avoiding alcohol becomes imperative, and dietary fat intake may need strict monitoring.
   - Regular medical check-ups and adherence to prescribed medications become part of the routine.

Navigating this diagnosis requires resilience, adaptability, and a willingness to embrace necessary changes. Support from healthcare professionals, peers, and loved ones is invaluable in fostering a positive outlook and empowering individuals to manage pancreatitis effectively.

Chapter 2: Building a Foundation for a Pancreatitis-Friendly Diet

Living well with pancreatitis involves more than just managing symptoms; it requires a fundamental shift in dietary choices. This chapter lays the groundwork for a pancreatitis-friendly diet, outlining key principles, highlighting foods to embrace, identifying those to avoid, and providing essential nutritional guidelines.

A. Key Principles of the Pancreatitis Diet:

1. Low Fat Intake:
   - Central to managing pancreatitis is the reduction of dietary fat. High-fat foods can trigger pancreatic inflammation and exacerbate symptoms.
   - Emphasis on choosing lean protein sources and incorporating healthy fats in moderation.

2. Small, Frequent Meals:
   - Opting for smaller, more frequent meals instead of large meals can help reduce the burden on the pancreas and ease digestion.
   - Snacking on nutritious, pancreatitis-friendly options between meals can maintain energy levels without overloading the digestive system.

3. Hydration:
   - Staying well-hydrated is crucial for overall health and aids in digestion.
   - Choosing water and herbal teas over sugary or caffeinated beverages helps prevent dehydration and supports pancreatic function.

4. Balanced Nutrition:
   - Striving for a well-balanced diet that includes a variety of nutrient-dense foods ensures that the body receives essential vitamins and minerals.
   - Focus on incorporating a colorful array of fruits, vegetables, whole grains, and lean proteins.

5. Individualized Approach:

- Recognizing that each individual's tolerance to specific foods varies, the pancreatitis diet may need to be personalized.
- Keeping a food journal and noting individual reactions can help identify trigger foods.

B. Foods to Embrace:

1. Lean Proteins:
- Skinless poultry, fish, tofu, and legumes are excellent sources of protein without excessive fat.
- Incorporating these proteins supports muscle health without overtaxing the pancreas.

2. Whole Grains:
- Quinoa, brown rice, and whole wheat products provide complex carbohydrates and fiber, promoting digestive health.
- These grains contribute to sustained energy levels without causing spikes in blood sugar.

3. Fruits and Vegetables:
- Opting for a variety of colorful fruits and vegetables ensures a diverse range of vitamins and antioxidants.
- Steaming or roasting vegetables can enhance flavor without the need for added fats.

4. Healthy Fats:
- Including sources of healthy fats, such as avocados, nuts, and olive oil, in moderation supports overall health.
- These fats can be incorporated mindfully to add flavor and nutritional value to meals.

C. Foods to Avoid:

1. High-Fat Foods:

- Fried foods, fatty cuts of meat, and full-fat dairy products should be limited or avoided.
- These items can contribute to inflammation and discomfort.

2. Processed and Sugary Foods:
   - Minimizing intake of processed foods and those high in added sugars helps maintain stable blood sugar levels.
   - Sugary treats and snacks may exacerbate inflammation and lead to unwanted weight gain.

3. Alcohol:
   - Given its impact on the pancreas, alcohol should be avoided or consumed in moderation.
   - Complete abstinence is often recommended, particularly in cases of chronic pancreatitis.

4. Spicy and Acidic Foods:
   - Spices and acidic foods may trigger digestive distress and should be approached with caution.
   - Monitoring individual tolerance to these items is essential.

D. Nutritional Guidelines:

1. Consult with a Registered Dietitian:
   - Seeking guidance from a registered dietitian can provide personalized advice based on individual health needs and preferences.
   - A dietitian can help create a balanced meal plan that aligns with nutritional goals and restrictions.

2. Monitor Nutrient Intake:
   - Paying attention to nutrient intake, particularly vitamins A, D, E, and K, helps prevent deficiencies associated with malabsorption.
   - Consider supplementation under the guidance of a healthcare professional.

3. Stay Informed on Pancreatic Enzyme Supplements:

- Some individuals with pancreatitis may benefit from pancreatic enzyme supplements to aid in digestion.
- Discussing the use of supplements with a healthcare provider is crucial for proper dosage and timing.

4. Gradual Introductions and Observation:
- When reintroducing foods or experimenting with new recipes, doing so gradually allows for the observation of any adverse reactions.
- Paying attention to the body's responses helps fine-tune the pancreatitis-friendly diet.

Building a foundation for a pancreatitis-friendly diet involves mindful choices, individualized adjustments, and a commitment to nourishing the body while respecting the constraints of the condition. The recipes and meal plans provided in this cookbook are crafted with these principles in mind, offering a delicious and nutritious approach to living well with pancreatitis.

Chapter 3: Essential Kitchen Tools and Ingredients

A. Kitchen Equipment for Easy Meal Preparation:

1. Blender:
   - Ideal for creating smoothies, purees, and soups. A blender can help you incorporate a variety of fruits and vegetables into your diet in an easily digestible form.

2. Food Processor:
   - Useful for chopping, dicing, and slicing fruits and vegetables. It's a versatile tool that can aid in the preparation of a wide range of pancreatitis-friendly recipes.

3. Steamer Basket:
   - Steaming vegetables is a gentle cooking method that helps retain nutrients while making them easy to digest. A steamer basket is a valuable addition to your kitchen.

4. Non-Stick Cookware:
   - Investing in non-stick pots and pans can reduce the need for excessive cooking oils, making it easier to adhere to a low-fat diet.

5. Sharp Knives:
   - High-quality, sharp knives make food preparation more efficient and safer. They are essential for cutting through a variety of fruits, vegetables, and lean proteins.

6. Slow Cooker or Instant Pot:
   - These appliances are excellent for preparing flavorful and tender meals with minimal effort. Slow cooking allows for the development of rich flavors without the need for excessive fat.

7. Measuring Cups and Spoons:
   - Precision in measuring ingredients is key, especially when following specific dietary guidelines. Having a set of measuring cups and spoons ensures accuracy in portion sizes.

8. Citrus Juicer:
   - Freshly squeezed citrus juices can add brightness and flavor to dishes without the need for excess fats. A citrus juicer makes it easy to incorporate this element into your cooking.

9. Digital Kitchen Scale:
   - Useful for accurately measuring ingredients, especially when it comes to portion control and maintaining a balanced diet.

10. Cutting Boards:
   - Having separate cutting boards for fruits, vegetables, and proteins helps prevent cross-contamination and ensures food safety.

B. Must-Have Pantry Staples:

1. Whole Grains:
   - Brown rice, quinoa, whole wheat pasta, and oats provide a nutritious base for meals, offering complex carbohydrates and fiber.

2. Canned Legumes:
   - Beans, lentils, and chickpeas are convenient protein sources that can be easily incorporated into salads, soups, and main dishes.

3. Low-Sodium Broth:
   - Vegetable or chicken broth serves as a flavorful base for soups and stews. Opt for low-sodium options to control salt intake.

4. Canned Tomatoes:
   - Diced or crushed tomatoes are versatile for sauces, soups, and stews. Choose varieties without added sugars or excessive sodium.

5. Healthy Oils:

 - Olive oil and avocado oil are heart-healthy fats that can be used in moderation for cooking and dressing salads.

6. Herbs and Spices:

 - Dried herbs and spices are essential for adding flavor without relying on excessive salt or fat. Consider having basil, oregano, thyme, cumin, and turmeric in your pantry.

7. Whole Grain Flour:

 - Whole wheat flour or alternative flours (such as almond or coconut flour) can be used for baking, providing a fiber-rich option.

8. Nuts and Seeds:

 - Almonds, walnuts, chia seeds, and flaxseeds are nutritious additions to meals, offering healthy fats and protein.

9. Nut Butters:

 - Natural peanut butter, almond butter, or other nut butters without added sugars or hydrogenated oils are excellent sources of protein and healthy fats.

10. Low-Fat Dairy or Dairy Alternatives:

 - Greek yogurt, skim milk, or plant-based alternatives like almond or soy milk can be used in recipes or enjoyed as snacks.

C. Fresh Ingredients to Enhance Flavor and Nutrition:

1. Leafy Greens:

 - Spinach, kale, and arugula are rich in vitamins and minerals. They can be incorporated into salads, smoothies, or sautéed as side dishes.

2. Colorful Vegetables:

 - Bell peppers, broccoli, carrots, and zucchini add variety, flavor, and essential nutrients to your meals.

3. Fresh Fruits:
   - Berries, apples, citrus fruits, and melons provide natural sweetness and a dose of vitamins. They can be enjoyed on their own or as part of recipes.

4. Lean Proteins:
   - Skinless poultry, fish, tofu, and legumes offer protein without excessive fat. Including a variety of these sources ensures a balanced diet.

5. Herbs and Citrus:
   - Fresh herbs like parsley, cilantro, and mint add freshness and depth to dishes. Citrus fruits (lemons, limes, oranges) can be used for zesting and juicing.

6. Garlic and Ginger:
   - These aromatic ingredients enhance the flavor of dishes without the need for excessive salt or fats.

7. Low-Fat Dairy:
   - Incorporating plain, low-fat yogurt or cottage cheese provides a creamy texture and additional protein to dishes.

8. Eggs:
   - A versatile protein source, eggs can be prepared in various ways to add nutrition to breakfast, lunch, or dinner.

9. Avocados:
   - Avocados contribute healthy fats and a creamy texture to dishes. They can be sliced, mashed, or added to salads.

10. Fresh Fish:
   - Fatty fish such as salmon or trout provide omega-3 fatty acids, supporting heart health. Include fish in your diet for a flavorful and nutritious option.

Chapter 4: Breakfasts

1. Berry and Banana Smoothie Bowl:

Ingredients:

- 1 cup mixed berries (strawberries, blueberries, raspberries)
- 1 ripe banana
- 1/2 cup low-fat Greek yogurt
- 1/4 cup rolled oats
- 1 tablespoon chia seeds
- 1/2 cup almond milk (unsweetened)
- 1 tablespoon honey (optional, for sweetness)
- Fresh mint leaves for garnish

Instructions:

1. In a blender, combine berries, banana, Greek yogurt, rolled oats, chia seeds, and almond milk.
2. Blend until smooth and creamy. If the mixture is too thick, you can add more almond milk as needed.
3. Pour the smoothie into a bowl.
4. Drizzle honey over the top for added sweetness (if desired).
5. Garnish with fresh mint leaves.
6. Enjoy with a spoon!

2. Veggie Omelette with Whole Grain Toast:

Ingredients:

- 2 large eggs
- 1/4 cup diced bell peppers (mixed colors)
- 1/4 cup diced tomatoes
- 1/4 cup diced onions
- 1/4 cup chopped spinach
- Salt and pepper to taste
- 1 teaspoon olive oil
- 2 slices whole grain bread, toasted

Instructions:

1. In a bowl, whisk the eggs and season with salt and pepper.

2. Heat olive oil in a non-stick skillet over medium heat.

3. Add bell peppers, tomatoes, onions, and spinach to the skillet. Sauté until vegetables are tender.

4. Pour the whisked eggs over the sautéed vegetables and cook until the edges set.

5. Carefully lift the edges of the omelette with a spatula to let the uncooked eggs flow underneath.

6. Once the eggs are mostly set, fold the omelette in half.

7. Slide the omelette onto a plate and serve with whole grain toast.

3. Banana-Oat Pancakes:

Ingredients:

- 1 ripe banana, mashed
- 2 large eggs
- 1/2 cup rolled oats
- 1/2 teaspoon baking powder
- 1/2 teaspoon vanilla extract
- Pinch of cinnamon (optional)
- Fresh fruit or berries for topping

Instructions:

1. In a bowl, combine mashed banana, eggs, rolled oats, baking powder, vanilla extract, and cinnamon.

2. Heat a non-stick skillet over medium heat.

3. Pour 1/4 cup of the batter onto the skillet to form each pancake.

4. Cook until bubbles form on the surface, then flip and cook the other side until golden brown.

5. Repeat with the remaining batter.

6. Serve the pancakes topped with fresh fruit or berries.

4. Greek Yogurt Parfait:

Ingredients:

- 1 cup low-fat Greek yogurt
- 1/2 cup mixed berries (strawberries, blueberries, raspberries)

- 1/4 cup granola (low-fat and low-sugar)
- 1 tablespoon honey
- 1 tablespoon chopped nuts (almonds, walnuts)

Instructions:
1. In a glass or bowl, layer Greek yogurt with mixed berries.
2. Sprinkle granola over the berries.
3. Drizzle honey on top.
4. Garnish with chopped nuts for added crunch.
5. Repeat the layering if desired.
6. Enjoy this satisfying and protein-packed parfait!

5. Spinach and Feta Breakfast Wrap:
Ingredients:
- 1 whole wheat or low-carb tortilla
- 2 large eggs, scrambled
- 1/2 cup fresh spinach leaves
- 2 tablespoons crumbled feta cheese
- Salt and pepper to taste
- 1 teaspoon olive oil

Instructions:
1. In a skillet, heat olive oil over medium heat.
2. Add fresh spinach and sauté until wilted.
3. Season scrambled eggs with salt and pepper, then add them to the skillet with spinach.
4. Stir until eggs are cooked through.
5. Place the egg and spinach mixture in the center of the tortilla.
6. Sprinkle feta cheese on top.
7. Fold the sides of the tortilla over the filling to create a wrap.
8. Heat in the skillet for a few minutes on each side until lightly browned.
9. Slice and serve this flavorful breakfast wrap.

6. Apple Cinnamon Overnight Oats:
Ingredients:
- 1/2 cup rolled oats
- 1/2 cup low-fat milk or a dairy-free alternative
- 1/2 cup unsweetened applesauce
- 1/2 teaspoon cinnamon
- 1 tablespoon chopped nuts (e.g., almonds, walnuts)
- Sliced apple for topping

Instructions:
1. In a jar or bowl, combine rolled oats, milk, applesauce, and cinnamon.
2. Stir well, ensuring oats are fully submerged in the liquid.
3. Cover and refrigerate overnight.
4. In the morning, give the oats a good stir.
5. Top with chopped nuts and sliced apple.
6. Enjoy this easy and nutritious grab-and-go breakfast.

7. Quinoa Breakfast Bowl:
Ingredients:
- 1/2 cup cooked quinoa
- 1/2 cup low-fat Greek yogurt
- 1/4 cup diced mango
- 1 tablespoon slivered almonds
- 1 teaspoon honey
- A dash of cinnamon

Instructions:
1. In a bowl, layer cooked quinoa and low-fat Greek yogurt.
2. Top with diced mango and slivered almonds.
3. Drizzle honey over the top.
4. Sprinkle it with a dash of cinnamon for added flavor.
5. Mix together before enjoying this protein-packed and satisfying breakfast bowl.

8. Smoked Salmon and Avocado Toast:
Ingredients:
- 1 slice whole grain bread, toasted
- 2 ounces smoked salmon
- 1/4 avocado, sliced
- 1 teaspoon capers
- Fresh dill for garnish
- Lemon wedges (optional)

Instructions:
1. Top the toasted bread with smoked salmon.
2. Arrange sliced avocado on top of the salmon.
3. Sprinkle capers over the avocado.
4. Garnish with fresh dill.
5. Serve with lemon wedges on the side for an extra burst of flavor.
6. This savory toast is a delightful and nutritious option.

9. Blueberry Almond Chia Pudding:
Ingredients:
- 2 tablespoons chia seeds
- 1/2 cup almond milk (unsweetened)
- 1/4 teaspoon almond extract
- 1/2 cup fresh blueberries
- 1 tablespoon sliced almonds
- 1 teaspoon honey (optional)

Instructions:
1. In a bowl, mix chia seeds, almond milk, and almond extract.
2. Let it sit in the refrigerator for at least 2 hours or overnight until it forms a pudding-like consistency.
3. Layer chia pudding with fresh blueberries.
4. Top with sliced almonds.
5. Drizzle with honey for sweetness if desired.
6. Enjoy this nutrient-packed and flavorful chia pudding.

10. Veggie Breakfast Burrito:
Ingredients:
- 1 whole wheat or low-carb tortilla
- 2 large eggs, scrambled
- 1/4 cup black beans, drained and rinsed
- 1/4 cup diced tomatoes
- 2 tablespoons diced red onion
- Salsa and cilantro for garnish

Instructions:
1. In a skillet, scramble the eggs until cooked through.
2. In the center of the tortilla, layer scrambled eggs, black beans, diced tomatoes, and red onion.
3. Roll the tortilla into a burrito.
4. Top with salsa and fresh cilantro.
5. Serve this protein-packed breakfast burrito for a savory start to the day.

11. Sweet Potato Breakfast Hash:
Ingredients:
- 1 medium sweet potato, peeled and grated
- 1/4 cup diced bell peppers (mixed colors)
- 1/4 cup diced red onion
- 1/4 cup black beans, drained and rinsed
- 2 large eggs
- 1 teaspoon olive oil
- Salt and pepper to taste
- Fresh cilantro for garnish

Instructions:
1. In a skillet, heat olive oil over medium heat.
2. Add grated sweet potato, bell peppers, and red onion. Sauté until sweet potato is tender.
3. Stir in black beans and cook until heated through.
4. Create wells in the hash and crack eggs into each well.
5. Cover the skillet and cook until the eggs are cooked to your liking.

6. Season with salt and pepper, garnish with fresh cilantro, and serve.

12. Cottage Cheese and Fruit Bowl:
Ingredients:
- 1/2 cup low-fat cottage cheese
- 1/2 cup diced pineapple
- 1/2 cup sliced strawberries
- 1/4 cup blueberries
- 1 tablespoon chopped walnuts
- Drizzle of honey (optional)

Instructions:
1. In a bowl, combine low-fat cottage cheese with diced pineapple, sliced strawberries, and blueberries.
2. Top with chopped walnuts for crunch.
3. Drizzle with honey if you desire additional sweetness.
4. Mix and enjoy this refreshing and protein-rich fruit bowl.

13. Turkey and Veggie Breakfast Wrap:
Ingredients:
- 1 whole wheat or low-carb tortilla
- 2 slices lean turkey breast
- 1/4 cup diced tomatoes
- 1/4 cup shredded lettuce
- 2 tablespoons salsa
- 1 tablespoon plain Greek yogurt

Instructions:
1. Lay turkey slices on the tortilla.
2. Top with diced tomatoes and shredded lettuce.
3. Spoon salsa and Greek yogurt over the veggies.
4. Roll into a wrap and serve.
5. This savory breakfast wrap is a protein-packed option.

14. Mango Coconut Chia Pudding:

Ingredients:

- 2 tablespoons chia seeds
- 1/2 cup coconut milk (unsweetened)
- 1/4 teaspoon vanilla extract
- 1/2 cup diced mango
- 1 tablespoon shredded coconut

Instructions:

1. In a bowl, mix chia seeds, coconut milk, and vanilla extract.
2. Refrigerate for at least 2 hours or overnight until it thickens.
3. Layer chia pudding with diced mango.
4. Sprinkle shredded coconut on top.
5. Enjoy this tropical and nutrient-rich chia pudding.

15. Vegetable and Egg Muffin Cups:

Ingredients:

- 4 large eggs
- 1/4 cup diced bell peppers (mixed colors)
- 1/4 cup diced zucchini
- 1/4 cup diced cherry tomatoes
- Salt and pepper to taste
- 2 tablespoons grated low-fat cheese (optional)

Instructions:

1. Preheat the oven to 350°F (175°C).
2. In a bowl, whisk eggs and season with salt and pepper.
3. Stir in diced bell peppers, zucchini, and cherry tomatoes.
4. Pour the mixture into greased muffin cups.
5. Top each cup with grated low-fat cheese if desired.
6. Bake for 15-20 minutes or until the eggs are set.
7. Allow to cool slightly before removing from the muffin tin.
8. These vegetable and egg muffin cups make for a convenient and portable breakfast.

16. Banana Walnut Oat Muffins:
Ingredients:
- 1 cup rolled oats
- 1/2 cup whole wheat flour
- 1/2 teaspoon baking soda
- 1/2 teaspoon baking powder
- 1/4 teaspoon salt
- 2 ripe bananas, mashed
- 1/4 cup honey
- 1/4 cup low-fat Greek yogurt
- 1 large egg
- 1/4 cup chopped walnuts

Instructions:
1. Preheat the oven to 375°F (190°C) and line a muffin tin with paper liners.
2. In a bowl, mix rolled oats, whole wheat flour, baking soda, baking powder, and salt.
3. In a separate bowl, whisk together mashed bananas, honey, Greek yogurt, and egg.
4. Add the wet ingredients to the dry ingredients and stir until just combined.
5. Fold in chopped walnuts.
6. Spoon the batter into muffin cups.
7. Bake for 18-20 minutes or until a toothpick comes out clean.
8. Allow muffins to cool before serving.

17. Tomato Basil Breakfast Quesadilla:
Ingredients:
- 1 whole wheat or low-carb tortilla
- 2 large eggs, scrambled
- 1/4 cup diced tomatoes
- 2 tablespoons chopped fresh basil
- 1/4 cup shredded low-fat mozzarella cheese
- Salt and pepper to taste

Instructions:

1. In a skillet, cook scrambled eggs until just set.

2. Place the tortilla in the skillet over low heat.

3. Spread scrambled eggs over half of the tortilla.

4. Top with diced tomatoes, fresh basil, and shredded mozzarella.

5. Fold the tortilla in half, pressing down with a spatula to seal.

6. Cook for a few minutes on each side until cheese is melted and tortilla is crispy.

7. Slice and serve this flavorful breakfast quesadilla.

18. Peanut Butter Banana Smoothie:

Ingredients:

- 1 ripe banana

- 2 tablespoons natural peanut butter

- 1/2 cup low-fat milk or a dairy-free alternative

- 1/2 cup low-fat Greek yogurt

- 1/2 cup ice cubes

- 1 tablespoon chia seeds (optional)

- Drizzle of honey (optional)

Instructions:

1. In a blender, combine ripe banana, peanut butter, low-fat milk, Greek yogurt, and ice cubes.

2. Blend until smooth and creamy.

3. Add chia seeds if desired and blend for a few seconds.

4. Drizzle honey over the top for added sweetness if needed.

5. Pour into a glass and enjoy this protein-packed smoothie.

19. Blueberry Lemon Muffins:

Ingredients:

- 1 cup whole wheat flour

- 1/2 cup rolled oats

- 1/2 teaspoon baking soda

- 1/2 teaspoon baking powder

- 1/4 teaspoon salt

- 1/4 cup melted coconut oil

- 1/4 cup honey
- 1/2 cup low-fat Greek yogurt
- 1 large egg
- 1 teaspoon vanilla extract
- Zest of one lemon
- 1 cup fresh or frozen blueberries

Instructions:
1. Preheat the oven to 350°F (175°C) and line a muffin tin with paper liners.
2. In a bowl, mix whole wheat flour, rolled oats, baking soda, baking powder, and salt.
3. In a separate bowl, whisk together melted coconut oil, honey, Greek yogurt, egg, vanilla extract, and lemon zest.
4. Add the wet ingredients to the dry ingredients and stir until just combined.
5. Gently fold in blueberries.
6. Spoon the batter into muffin cups.
7. Bake for 18-20 minutes or until a toothpick comes out clean.
8. Allow muffins to cool before serving.

20. Veggie and Feta Egg Muffins:
Ingredients:
- 6 large eggs
- 1/4 cup diced bell peppers (mixed colors)
- 1/4 cup diced zucchini
- 1/4 cup cherry tomatoes, halved
- 2 tablespoons crumbled feta cheese
- Salt and pepper to taste
- Fresh parsley for garnish

Instructions:
1. Preheat the oven to 350°F (175°C) and grease a muffin tin.
2. In a bowl, whisk eggs and season with salt and pepper.
3. Distribute diced bell peppers, zucchini, and cherry tomatoes evenly among the muffin cups.
4. Pour the whisked eggs over the vegetables in each cup.

5. Top with crumbled feta cheese.
6. Bake for 15-20 minutes or until the eggs are set.
7. Garnish with fresh parsley and serve.

Chapter 5: Satisfying Snacks

1. Greek Yogurt with Berries:
Ingredients:
- 1 cup low-fat Greek yogurt
- 1/2 cup mixed berries (strawberries, blueberries, raspberries)

Instructions:
1. In a bowl, spoon low-fat Greek yogurt.
2. Top with mixed berries.
3. Mix gently and enjoy.

2. Veggie Sticks with Hummus:
Ingredients:
- Assorted veggie sticks (carrots, cucumbers, bell peppers)
- 1/4 cup low-fat hummus

Instructions:
1. Slice vegetables into sticks.
2. Serve with a side of low-fat hummus.
3. Dip and enjoy!

3. Apple Slices with Peanut Butter:
Ingredients:
- 1 apple, sliced
- 2 tablespoons natural peanut butter

Instructions:
1. Slice the apple into wedges.
2. Spread peanut butter on each slice.
3. Enjoy this sweet and savory combo.

4. Rice Cakes with Cottage Cheese:
Ingredients:
- Whole grain rice cakes

- 1/2 cup low-fat cottage cheese

Instructions:
1. Spread low-fat cottage cheese on rice cakes.
2. Enjoy this light and protein-filled snack.

5. Mixed Nuts and Dried Fruit:
Ingredients:
- 1/4 cup mixed unsalted nuts
- 1/4 cup dried fruits (raisins, apricots, cranberries)

Instructions:
1. Combine mixed nuts and dried fruits in a bowl.
2. Toss together and enjoy this energy-boosting mix.

6. Whole Grain Crackers with Tuna Salad:
Ingredients:
- Whole grain crackers
- 1/2 cup canned tuna, drained
- 1 tablespoon low-fat mayonnaise or Greek yogurt
- Salt and pepper to taste

Instructions:
1. Mix tuna with low-fat mayo or Greek yogurt.
2. Spoon tuna salad onto whole grain crackers.
3. Enjoy this satisfying and protein-packed snack.

7. Roasted Chickpeas:
Ingredients:
- 1 cup canned chickpeas, drained and rinsed
- 1 tablespoon olive oil
- 1/2 teaspoon paprika
- 1/2 teaspoon cumin
- Salt to taste

Instructions:
1. Preheat the oven to 400°F (200°C).
2. Toss chickpeas with olive oil, paprika, cumin, and salt.
3. Roast for 20-25 minutes until crispy.
4. Allow to cool before enjoying.

8. Cottage Cheese and Pineapple Cubes:
Ingredients:
- 1/2 cup low-fat cottage cheese
- 1/2 cup fresh pineapple, cubed

Instructions:
1. Spoon low-fat cottage cheese into a bowl.
2. Top with fresh pineapple cubes.
3. Mix and enjoy this refreshing snack.

9. Edamame Pods:
Ingredients:
- 1 cup edamame pods
- Sea salt to taste

Instructions:
1. Steam or boil edamame pods until tender.
2. Sprinkle with sea salt.
3. Enjoy this protein-packed and satisfying snack.

10. Veggie Wrap:
Ingredients:
- Whole wheat wrap
- Sliced cucumber, bell peppers, cherry tomatoes
- 2 tablespoons hummus

Instructions:
1. Lay out a whole wheat wrap.
2. Spread hummus over the wrap.

3. Add sliced veggies and roll into a wrap.
4. Slice and enjoy!

11. Hard-Boiled Eggs:
Ingredients:
- 2 hard-boiled eggs
- Salt and pepper to taste

Instructions:
1. Peel hard-boiled eggs.
2. Sprinkle with salt and pepper.
3. Enjoy this quick and protein-rich snack.

12. Low-Fat Yogurt Parfait:
Ingredients:
- 1 cup low-fat yogurt
- 1/4 cup granola
- 1/2 cup mixed berries (strawberries, blueberries)

Instructions:
1. In a glass, layer low-fat yogurt with granola and mixed berries.
2. Repeat the layers.
3. Enjoy this parfait that's both delicious and nutritious.

13. Sliced Avocado on Rice Cakes:
Ingredients:
- Whole grain rice cakes
- 1/2 avocado, sliced
- Salt and pepper to taste

Instructions:
1. Spread avocado slices on rice cakes.
2. Season with salt and pepper.
3. Enjoy this creamy and nutrient-dense snack.

14. Cherry Tomatoes with Balsamic Glaze:
Ingredients:
- Cherry tomatoes
- Balsamic glaze

Instructions:
1. Arrange cherry tomatoes on a plate.
2. Drizzle with balsamic glaze.
3. Enjoy this sweet and tangy snack.

15. Air-Popped Popcorn:
Ingredients:
- 1/2 cup air-popped popcorn
- Nutritional yeast to taste

Instructions:
1. Pop the popcorn using an air popper.
2. Sprinkle with nutritional yeast.
3. Enjoy this low-fat and savory treat.

16. Banana and Almond Butter:
Ingredients:
- 1 banana, sliced
- 2 tablespoons almond butter

Instructions:
1. Slice the banana.
2. Spread almond butter on each slice.
3. Enjoy this satisfying and potassium-rich snack.

17. Low-Fat Cheese Cubes:
Ingredients:
- Low-fat cheese cubes
- Whole grain crackers

Instructions:
1. Arrange low-fat cheese cubes on a plate.
2. Serve with whole grain crackers.
3. Enjoy this quick and protein-rich snack.

18. Celery Sticks with Peanut Butter:
Ingredients:
- Celery sticks
- 2 tablespoons natural peanut butter

Instructions:
1. Spread peanut butter inside celery sticks.
2. Enjoy this crunchy and satisfying snack.

19. Berries and Cottage Cheese Bowl:
Ingredients:
- 1/2 cup low-fat cottage cheese
- 1/2 cup mixed berries (strawberries, blueberries)

Instructions:
1. Spoon low-fat cottage cheese into a bowl.
2. Top with mixed berries.
3. Mix and enjoy this sweet and protein-packed snack.

20. Sliced Peaches with Yogurt:
Ingredients:
- 1 peach, sliced
- 1/2 cup low-fat yogurt

Instructions:
1. Arrange peach slices on a plate.
2. Serve with a side of low-fat yogurt.
3. Enjoy this refreshing and vitamin-rich snack.

Chapter 6: Soups and Salads

1. Minestrone Soup:
Ingredients:
- 1 tablespoon olive oil
- 1 onion, diced
- 2 carrots, diced
- 2 celery stalks, diced
- 2 cloves garlic, minced
- 1 can (15 oz) kidney beans, drained and rinsed
- 1 can (15 oz) diced tomatoes
- 4 cups vegetable broth
- 1 cup green beans, chopped
- 1 cup whole wheat pasta
- 1 teaspoon dried oregano
- 1 teaspoon dried basil
- Salt and pepper to taste
- Fresh parsley for garnish

Instructions:
1. In a large pot, heat olive oil over medium heat.
2. Add diced onion, carrots, and celery. Cook until vegetables are softened.
3. Add minced garlic and cook for an additional minute.
4. Pour in diced tomatoes, kidney beans, vegetable broth, green beans, pasta, oregano, and basil.
5. Season with salt and pepper to taste.
6. Bring to a boil, then reduce heat and simmer until pasta is cooked.
7. Garnish with fresh parsley before serving.

2. Greek Salad:
Ingredients:
- 2 cups cherry tomatoes, halved
- 1 cucumber, diced
- 1 bell pepper, diced
- 1/2 red onion, thinly sliced

- 1 cup Kalamata olives, pitted
- 1 cup feta cheese, crumbled
- 1/4 cup extra-virgin olive oil
- 2 tablespoons red wine vinegar
- 1 teaspoon dried oregano
- Salt and pepper to taste

Instructions:
1. In a large bowl, combine cherry tomatoes, cucumber, bell pepper, red onion, olives, and feta cheese.
2. In a small bowl, whisk together olive oil, red wine vinegar, dried oregano, salt, and pepper.
3. Pour the dressing over the salad and toss gently to combine.
4. Refrigerate for at least 30 minutes before serving.

3. Lentil Soup:
Ingredients:
- 1 tablespoon olive oil
- 1 onion, diced
- 2 carrots, diced
- 2 celery stalks, diced
- 2 cloves garlic, minced
- 1 cup dry lentils, rinsed and drained
- 4 cups vegetable broth
- 1 can (15 oz) diced tomatoes
- 1 teaspoon ground cumin
- 1 teaspoon ground coriander
- 1/2 teaspoon smoked paprika
- Salt and pepper to taste
- Fresh cilantro for garnish

Instructions:
1. In a large pot, heat olive oil over medium heat.
2. Add diced onion, carrots, and celery. Cook until vegetables are softened.
3. Add minced garlic and cook for an additional minute.

4. Stir in lentils, vegetable broth, diced tomatoes, cumin, coriander, smoked paprika, salt, and pepper.
5. Bring to a boil, then reduce heat and simmer until lentils are tender.
6. Garnish with fresh cilantro before serving.

4. Caesar Salad:
Ingredients:
- 1 head romaine lettuce, chopped
- 1/2 cup croutons (whole wheat for a healthier option)
- 1/4 cup grated Parmesan cheese
- 1/4 cup low-fat Caesar dressing
- 1 tablespoon lemon juice
- 1 teaspoon Dijon mustard
- Salt and pepper to taste

Instructions:
1. In a large bowl, combine chopped romaine lettuce and croutons.
2. In a small bowl, whisk together Parmesan cheese, Caesar dressing, lemon juice, Dijon mustard, salt, and pepper.
3. Pour the dressing over the salad and toss gently to coat.
4. Serve immediately.

5. Tomato Basil Soup:
Ingredients:
- 1 tablespoon olive oil
- 1 onion, diced
- 2 cloves garlic, minced
- 1 can (28 oz) crushed tomatoes
- 1 can (14 oz) vegetable broth
- 1 teaspoon dried basil
- 1/2 teaspoon dried oregano
- Salt and pepper to taste
- 1/4 cup fresh basil, chopped (for garnish)
- 1/4 cup low-fat Greek yogurt (optional, for garnish)

Instructions:
1. In a large pot, heat olive oil over medium heat.
2. Add diced onion and cook until softened.
3. Add minced garlic and cook for an additional minute.
4. Stir in crushed tomatoes, vegetable broth, dried basil, dried oregano, salt, and pepper.
5. Bring to a simmer and let it cook for about 15-20 minutes.
6. Use an immersion blender to blend the soup until smooth.
7. Garnish with fresh basil and a dollop of low-fat Greek yogurt if desired.

6. Butternut Squash Soup:
Ingredients:
- 1 butternut squash, peeled and diced
- 1 onion, diced
- 2 carrots, diced
- 2 apples, peeled and chopped
- 4 cups vegetable broth
- 1 teaspoon ground cinnamon
- 1/2 teaspoon nutmeg
- Salt and pepper to taste
- 2 tablespoons low-fat Greek yogurt (for garnish)

Instructions:
1. In a large pot, sauté onions until softened.
2. Add butternut squash, carrots, apples, vegetable broth, cinnamon, nutmeg, salt, and pepper.
3. Bring to a boil, then simmer until vegetables are tender.
4. Use a blender to puree the soup until smooth.
5. Garnish with a dollop of low-fat Greek yogurt before serving.

7. Spinach and Strawberry Salad:
Ingredients:
- 4 cups baby spinach
- 1 cup strawberries, sliced
- 1/4 cup red onion, thinly sliced

- 1/4 cup feta cheese, crumbled
- 2 tablespoons balsamic vinaigrette dressing

Instructions:
1. In a large bowl, combine baby spinach, sliced strawberries, red onion, and feta cheese.
2. Drizzle with balsamic vinaigrette dressing.
3. Toss gently to coat the salad evenly.
4. Serve immediately.

8. Black Bean Soup:
Ingredients:
- 1 tablespoon olive oil
- 1 onion, diced
- 2 cloves garlic, minced
- 2 cans (15 oz each) black beans, drained and rinsed
- 1 can (14 oz) vegetable broth
- 1 can (14 oz) diced tomatoes
- 1 teaspoon ground cumin
- 1 teaspoon chili powder
- Salt and pepper to taste
- Fresh cilantro for garnish

Instructions:
1. In a large pot, heat olive oil over medium heat.
2. Add diced onions and sauté until translucent.
3. Add minced garlic and cook for an additional minute.
4. Stir in black beans, vegetable broth, diced tomatoes, cumin, chili powder, salt, and pepper.
5. Bring to a simmer and let it cook for about 15-20 minutes.
6. Garnish with fresh cilantro before serving.

9. Quinoa Salad with Lemon Vinaigrette:
Ingredients:
- 1 cup cooked quinoa

- 1 cucumber, diced
- 1 bell pepper, diced
- 1 cup cherry tomatoes, halved
- 1/4 cup red onion, finely chopped
- 1/4 cup feta cheese, crumbled
- 2 tablespoons olive oil
- 2 tablespoons lemon juice
- 1 teaspoon Dijon mustard
- Salt and pepper to taste

Instructions:
1. In a large bowl, combine cooked quinoa, cucumber, bell pepper, cherry tomatoes, red onion, and feta cheese.
2. In a small bowl, whisk together olive oil, lemon juice, Dijon mustard, salt, and pepper.
3. Pour the dressing over the salad and toss gently to combine.
4. Refrigerate for at least 30 minutes before serving.

10. Chicken and Vegetable Soup:
Ingredients:
- 1 tablespoon olive oil
- 1 onion, diced
- 2 carrots, diced
- 2 celery stalks, diced
- 2 cloves garlic, minced
- 1 pound boneless, skinless chicken breast, diced
- 4 cups chicken broth
- 1 cup broccoli florets
- 1 cup cauliflower florets
- 1 teaspoon dried thyme
- Salt and pepper to taste
- Fresh parsley for garnish

Instructions:
1. In a large pot, heat olive oil over medium heat.

2. Add diced onion, carrots, celery, and garlic. Cook until vegetables are softened.
3. Add diced chicken and cook until browned.
4. Pour in chicken broth, broccoli, cauliflower, dried thyme, salt, and pepper.
5. Bring to a boil, then reduce heat and simmer until chicken is cooked through.
6. Garnish with fresh parsley before serving.

11. Sweet Potato and Lentil Soup:
Ingredients:
- 1 tablespoon olive oil
- 1 onion, diced
- 2 cloves garlic, minced
- 2 sweet potatoes, peeled and diced
- 1 cup dry lentils, rinsed and drained
- 6 cups vegetable broth
- 1 teaspoon ground cumin
- 1/2 teaspoon smoked paprika
- Salt and pepper to taste
- Fresh cilantro for garnish

Instructions:
1. In a large pot, heat olive oil over medium heat.
2. Add diced onions and cook until softened.
3. Add minced garlic and cook for an additional minute.
4. Stir in sweet potatoes, lentils, vegetable broth, ground cumin, smoked paprika, salt, and pepper.
5. Bring to a boil, then reduce heat and simmer until sweet potatoes and lentils are tender.
6. Garnish with fresh cilantro before serving.

12. Caprese Salad:
Ingredients:
- 2 cups cherry tomatoes, halved
- 1 cup fresh mozzarella balls
- 1/4 cup fresh basil leaves, torn
- 2 tablespoons balsamic glaze

- 1 tablespoon extra-virgin olive oil
- Salt and pepper to taste

Instructions:
1. In a serving bowl, combine cherry tomatoes, fresh mozzarella balls, and torn basil leaves.
2. Drizzle with balsamic glaze and olive oil.
3. Season with salt and pepper to taste.
4. Gently toss and serve.

13. Vegetable Barley Soup:
Ingredients:
- 1 tablespoon olive oil
- 1 onion, diced
- 2 carrots, diced
- 2 celery stalks, diced
- 2 cloves garlic, minced
- 1 cup pearl barley, rinsed and drained
- 6 cups vegetable broth
- 1 cup green beans, chopped
- 1 cup corn kernels
- 1 teaspoon dried thyme
- Salt and pepper to taste
- Fresh parsley for garnish

Instructions:
1. In a large pot, heat olive oil over medium heat.
2. Add diced onions, carrots, celery, and garlic. Cook until vegetables are softened.
3. Stir in pearl barley, vegetable broth, green beans, corn, dried thyme, salt, and pepper.
4. Bring to a boil, then reduce heat and simmer until barley is cooked.
5. Garnish with fresh parsley before serving.

14. Tuna Salad Lettuce Wraps:
Ingredients:
- 1 can (5 oz) tuna, drained
- 1/4 cup low-fat Greek yogurt
- 1 tablespoon Dijon mustard
- 2 tablespoons red onion, finely chopped
- 2 tablespoons celery, finely chopped
- Salt and pepper to taste
- Lettuce leaves for wrapping

Instructions:
1. In a bowl, mix tuna, Greek yogurt, Dijon mustard, red onion, celery, salt, and pepper.
2. Spoon the tuna mixture onto lettuce leaves.
3. Roll into wraps and enjoy this light and protein-rich meal.

15. Tomato and White Bean Soup:
Ingredients:
- 1 tablespoon olive oil
- 1 onion, diced
- 2 cloves garlic, minced
- 2 cans (15 oz each) white beans, drained and rinsed
- 1 can (14 oz) diced tomatoes
- 4 cups vegetable broth
- 1 teaspoon dried rosemary
- 1 teaspoon dried thyme
- Salt and pepper to taste
- Fresh basil for garnish

Instructions:
1. In a large pot, heat olive oil over medium heat.
2. Add diced onions and cook until softened.
3. Add minced garlic and cook for an additional minute.
4. Stir in white beans, diced tomatoes, vegetable broth, dried rosemary, dried thyme, salt, and pepper.

5. Bring to a simmer and let it cook for about 15-20 minutes.
6. Garnish with fresh basil before serving.

16. Caesar Chickpea Salad:
Ingredients:
- 1 can (15 oz) chickpeas, drained and rinsed
- 1 tablespoon olive oil
- 1 teaspoon garlic powder
- 1/4 cup grated Parmesan cheese
- 4 cups romaine lettuce, chopped
- 1/4 cup croutons (whole wheat for a healthier option)
- 1/4 cup low-fat Caesar dressing

Instructions:
1. In a skillet, heat olive oil over medium heat.
2. Add chickpeas, garlic powder, and grated Parmesan. Cook until chickpeas are crispy.
3. In a large bowl, combine chopped romaine lettuce, croutons, and the crispy chickpeas.
4. Drizzle with low-fat Caesar dressing and toss gently.
5. Serve immediately.

17. Broccoli and Cheddar Soup:
Ingredients:
- 1 tablespoon olive oil
- 1 onion, diced
- 2 cloves garlic, minced
- 4 cups broccoli florets
- 4 cups vegetable broth
- 1 cup low-fat cheddar cheese, shredded
- 1 cup low-fat milk
- Salt and pepper to taste
- Nutmeg for garnish (optional)

Instructions:

1. In a large pot, heat olive oil over medium heat.
2. Add diced onions and cook until softened.
3. Add minced garlic and cook for an additional minute.
4. Stir in broccoli, vegetable broth, low-fat cheddar cheese, low-fat milk, salt, and pepper.
5. Bring to a boil, then reduce heat and simmer until broccoli is tender.
6. Use an immersion blender to blend the soup until smooth.
7. Garnish with a pinch of nutmeg if desired.

18. Grilled Chicken Salad:

Ingredients:

- 1 boneless, skinless chicken breast
- 1 tablespoon olive oil
- 1 teaspoon dried Italian seasoning
- Salt and pepper to taste
- 4 cups mixed salad greens
- 1 cup cherry tomatoes, halved
- 1/2 cucumber, sliced
- 1/4 cup balsamic vinaigrette dressing

Instructions:

1. Season chicken breast with olive oil, Italian seasoning, salt, and pepper.
2. Grill the chicken until cooked through.
3. Slice the grilled chicken into strips.
4. In a large bowl, combine mixed salad greens, cherry tomatoes, cucumber, and grilled chicken.
5. Drizzle with balsamic vinaigrette dressing and toss gently.
6. Serve immediately.

19. Vegetable Noodle Soup:

Ingredients:

- 1 tablespoon olive oil
- 1 onion, diced
- 2 carrots, julienned

- 2 celery stalks, sliced
- 2 cloves garlic, minced
- 4 cups vegetable broth
- 2 cups spiralized zucchini noodles
- 1 cup spinach leaves
- 1 teaspoon dried thyme
- Salt and pepper to taste
- Fresh dill for garnish

Instructions:
1. In a large pot, heat olive oil over medium heat.
2. Add diced onions, julienned carrots, sliced celery, and minced garlic. Cook until vegetables are softened.
3. Pour in vegetable broth, zucchini noodles, spinach, dried thyme, salt, and pepper.
4. Bring to a boil, then reduce heat and simmer until noodles are tender.
5. Garnish with fresh dill before serving.

20. Waldorf Chicken Salad:
Ingredients:
- 1 cup cooked and shredded chicken breast
- 1/2 cup celery, diced
- 1/2 cup red grapes, halved
- 1/4 cup walnuts, chopped
- 1/4 cup low-fat mayonnaise
- 1 tablespoon Greek yogurt
- 1 tablespoon lemon juice
- Salt and pepper to taste
- Butter lettuce leaves for serving

Instructions:
1. In a bowl, combine shredded chicken, diced celery, halved red grapes, and chopped walnuts.
2. In a separate bowl, whisk together low-fat mayonnaise, Greek yogurt, lemon juice, salt, and pepper.

3. Pour the dressing over the chicken mixture and toss gently.
4. Spoon the Waldorf chicken salad into butter lettuce leaves.
5. Serve and enjoy this refreshing and protein-packed salad.

Chapter 7: Main Courses

1. Grilled Lemon Herb Chicken:
Ingredients:
- 4 boneless, skinless chicken breasts
- 2 tablespoons olive oil
- 1 tablespoon lemon juice
- 1 teaspoon dried thyme
- 1 teaspoon dried rosemary
- Salt and pepper to taste

Instructions:
1. Preheat grill to medium-high heat.
2. In a bowl, mix olive oil, lemon juice, dried thyme, dried rosemary, salt, and pepper.
3. Coat chicken breasts with the marinade.
4. Grill chicken for 6-8 minutes per side or until cooked through.

2. Baked Salmon with Dill Sauce:
Ingredients:
- 4 salmon fillets
- 2 tablespoons olive oil
- 1 tablespoon lemon juice
- 2 tablespoons fresh dill, chopped
- Salt and pepper to taste

Instructions:
1. Preheat oven to 375°F (190°C).
2. Place salmon fillets on a baking sheet.
3. Mix olive oil, lemon juice, fresh dill, salt, and pepper.
4. Brush the salmon with the mixture.
5. Bake for 15-20 minutes or until the salmon is cooked through.

3. Turkey and Vegetable Stir-Fry:
Ingredients:
- 1 pound lean ground turkey
- 2 tablespoons low-sodium soy sauce
- 1 tablespoon olive oil
- 1 bell pepper, sliced
- 1 cup broccoli florets
- 1 carrot, julienned
- 2 cloves garlic, minced

Instructions:
1. In a skillet, cook ground turkey with olive oil until browned.
2. Add soy sauce, bell pepper, broccoli, carrot, and garlic.
3. Stir-fry until vegetables are tender.

4. Shrimp and Veggie Skewers:
Ingredients:
- 1 pound shrimp, peeled and deveined
- 2 tablespoons olive oil
- 1 tablespoon lemon juice
- 1 teaspoon paprika
- 1 zucchini, sliced
- 1 red onion, sliced
- Cherry tomatoes

Instructions:
1. Preheat grill to medium-high heat.
2. In a bowl, mix olive oil, lemon juice, and paprika.
3. Thread shrimp, zucchini, red onion, and cherry tomatoes onto skewers.
4. Grill for 2-3 minutes per side or until shrimp is cooked.

5. Quinoa-Stuffed Peppers:
Ingredients:
- 4 bell peppers, halved and seeded
- 1 cup quinoa, cooked

- 1 can (15 oz) black beans, drained and rinsed
- 1 cup corn kernels
- 1 cup salsa
- 1 teaspoon cumin
- Salt and pepper to taste

Instructions:
1. Preheat oven to 375°F (190°C).
2. In a bowl, mix cooked quinoa, black beans, corn, salsa, cumin, salt, and pepper.
3. Stuff bell peppers with the quinoa mixture.
4. Bake for 25-30 minutes or until peppers are tender.

6. Lemon Garlic Tilapia:
Ingredients:
- 4 tilapia fillets
- 2 tablespoons olive oil
- 2 tablespoons lemon juice
- 3 cloves garlic, minced
- 1 teaspoon dried oregano
- Salt and pepper to taste

Instructions:
1. Preheat oven to 400°F (200°C).
2. Place tilapia fillets on a baking sheet.
3. Mix olive oil, lemon juice, minced garlic, dried oregano, salt, and pepper.
4. Drizzle the mixture over the tilapia.
5. Bake for 12-15 minutes or until fish flakes easily.

7. Chickpea and Spinach Curry:
Ingredients:
- 2 cans (15 oz each) chickpeas, drained and rinsed
- 1 tablespoon olive oil
- 1 onion, diced
- 2 cloves garlic, minced
- 1 tablespoon curry powder

- 1 can (14 oz) diced tomatoes
- 4 cups baby spinach
- Salt and pepper to taste

Instructions:
1. In a skillet, heat olive oil over medium heat.
2. Add diced onions and cook until softened.
3. Add minced garlic and curry powder. Cook for 1 minute.
4. Stir in chickpeas, diced tomatoes, baby spinach, salt, and pepper.
5. Simmer until spinach is wilted.

8. Baked Chicken Parmesan:
Ingredients:
- 4 boneless, skinless chicken breasts
- 1 cup whole wheat breadcrumbs
- 1/2 cup grated Parmesan cheese
- 1 teaspoon dried oregano
- 1 cup marinara sauce
- 1 cup part-skim mozzarella cheese

Instructions:
1. Preheat oven to 400°F (200°C).
2. In a bowl, mix breadcrumbs, Parmesan, and dried oregano.
3. Dip chicken breasts into the breadcrumb mixture.
4. Place chicken on a baking sheet and bake for 20 minutes.
5. Spoon marinara sauce over each chicken breast and top with mozzarella.
6. Bake for an additional 10-15 minutes or until chicken is cooked through.

9. Veggie and Tofu Stir-Fry:
Ingredients:
- 1 block firm tofu, pressed and cubed
- 2 tablespoons low-sodium soy sauce
- 1 tablespoon sesame oil
- 1 tablespoon rice vinegar
- 1 tablespoon honey

- 1 tablespoon olive oil
- Assorted vegetables (broccoli, bell peppers, snap peas)

Instructions:
1. In a bowl, mix soy sauce, sesame oil, rice vinegar, and honey.
2. In a skillet, heat olive oil over medium heat.
3. Add cubed tofu and stir-fry until golden brown.
4. Add assorted vegetables and sauce mixture. Stir-fry until vegetables are tender.

10. Mediterranean Baked Cod:
Ingredients:
- 4 cod fillets
- 2 tablespoons olive oil
- 1 tablespoon lemon juice
- 2 cloves garlic, minced
- 1 teaspoon dried oregano
- 1 cup cherry tomatoes, halved
- 1/4 cup Kalamata olives, sliced
- 1/4 cup feta cheese, crumbled

Instructions:
1. Preheat oven to 400°F (200°C).
2. Place cod fillets on a baking sheet.
3. Mix olive oil, lemon juice, minced garlic, and dried oregano.
4. Drizzle the mixture over the cod.
5. Top with cherry tomatoes, Kalamata olives, and feta.
6. Bake for 15-20 minutes or until fish is cooked through.

11. Sweet and Sour Chicken:
Ingredients:
- 1 pound boneless, skinless chicken breast, diced
- 1 cup pineapple chunks
- 1 bell pepper, diced
- 1 onion, diced
- 1/4 cup low-sodium soy sauce

- 1/4 cup rice vinegar
- 2 tablespoons honey
- 1 tablespoon cornstarch
- 1 tablespoon olive oil

Instructions:
1. In a bowl, mix soy sauce, rice vinegar, honey, and cornstarch.
2. In a skillet, heat olive oil over medium heat.
3. Add diced chicken and cook until browned.
4. Add pineapple chunks, bell pepper, and onion. Cook until vegetables are tender.
5. Pour the sauce over the chicken and vegetables. Stir until the sauce thickens.

12. Spaghetti Squash with Turkey Bolognese:
Ingredients:
- 1 medium spaghetti squash, halved and seeded
- 1 pound lean ground turkey
- 1 can (14 oz) diced tomatoes
- 1/4 cup tomato paste
- 2 cloves garlic, minced
- 1 teaspoon dried basil
- 1 teaspoon dried oregano
- Salt and pepper to taste
- Fresh parsley for garnish

Instructions:
1. Preheat oven to 400°F (200°C).
2. Place spaghetti squash halves on a baking sheet, cut side down.
3. Roast for 40-45 minutes or until tender.
4. In a skillet, cook ground turkey until browned.
5. Add diced tomatoes, tomato paste, minced garlic, dried basil, dried oregano, salt, and pepper.
6. Simmer until the sauce thickens.
7. Use a fork to scrape the spaghetti squash into "noodles."
8. Top with turkey bolognese and garnish with fresh parsley.

13. Lemon Garlic Shrimp and Asparagus:
Ingredients:
- 1 pound shrimp, peeled and deveined
- 1 bunch asparagus, trimmed
- 2 tablespoons olive oil
- 2 tablespoons lemon juice
- 3 cloves garlic, minced
- 1 teaspoon dried thyme
- Salt and pepper to taste

Instructions:
1. Preheat oven to 400°F (200°C).
2. Place shrimp and asparagus on a baking sheet.
3. In a bowl, mix olive oil, lemon juice, minced garlic, dried thyme, salt, and pepper.
4. Drizzle the mixture over shrimp and asparagus.
5. Bake for 10-12 minutes or until shrimp is cooked and asparagus is tender.

14. Veggie-Packed Turkey Chili:
Ingredients:
- 1 pound lean ground turkey
- 1 onion, diced
- 2 cloves garlic, minced
- 1 bell pepper, diced
- 1 zucchini, diced
- 1 can (14 oz) diced tomatoes
- 1 can (15 oz) kidney beans, drained and rinsed
- 2 tablespoons chili powder
- 1 teaspoon cumin
- Salt and pepper to taste

Instructions:
1. In a large pot, cook ground turkey until browned.
2. Add diced onions, minced garlic, bell pepper, and zucchini. Cook until vegetables are tender.

3. Stir in diced tomatoes, kidney beans, chili powder, cumin, salt, and pepper.
4. Simmer for 20-30 minutes.

15. Teriyaki Tofu and Broccoli:
Ingredients:
- 1 block extra-firm tofu, pressed and cubed
- 2 tablespoonslow-sodium teriyaki sauce
- 1 tablespoon olive oil
- 2 tablespoons low-sodium soy sauce
- 1 tablespoon rice vinegar
- 1 tablespoon honey
- 2 cups broccoli florets

Instructions:
1. In a bowl, combine tofu cubes with teriyaki sauce. Let it marinate for at least 15 minutes.
2. In a skillet, heat olive oil over medium heat.
3. Add marinated tofu cubes and cook until golden brown.
4. In a separate bowl, mix soy sauce, rice vinegar, and honey.
5. Add broccoli to the skillet and pour the soy sauce mixture over tofu and broccoli.
6. Stir-fry until the broccoli is tender.

16. Eggplant and Chickpea Tagine:
Ingredients:
- 1 eggplant, diced
- 1 can (15 oz) chickpeas, drained and rinsed
- 1 onion, diced
- 2 cloves garlic, minced
- 1 can (14 oz) diced tomatoes
- 1 teaspoon ground cumin
- 1 teaspoon ground coriander
- 1/2 teaspoon cinnamon
- Salt and pepper to taste
- Fresh cilantro for garnish

Instructions:
1. In a large pot, sauté diced onions until softened.
2. Add minced garlic and cook for an additional minute.
3. Add diced eggplant, chickpeas, diced tomatoes, ground cumin, ground coriander, cinnamon, salt, and pepper.
4. Simmer until the eggplant is tender.
5. Garnish with fresh cilantro before serving.

17. Chicken and Broccoli Stir-Fry:
Ingredients:
- 1 pound boneless, skinless chicken breast, thinly sliced
- 2 tablespoons low-sodium soy sauce
- 1 tablespoon olive oil
- 2 cloves garlic, minced
- 1 teaspoon fresh ginger, grated
- 2 cups broccoli florets
- 1 carrot, julienned

Instructions:
1. In a bowl, marinate chicken slices with soy sauce.
2. In a wok or skillet, heat olive oil over medium-high heat.
3. Add minced garlic and grated ginger. Stir-fry for 1 minute.
4. Add marinated chicken and cook until browned.
5. Stir in broccoli florets and julienned carrots. Cook until vegetables are tender.

18. Quinoa and Black Bean Stuffed Peppers:
Ingredients:
- 4 bell peppers, halved and seeded
- 1 cup quinoa, cooked
- 1 can (15 oz) black beans, drained and rinsed
- 1 cup corn kernels
- 1 cup salsa
- 1 teaspoon cumin
- Salt and pepper to taste
- Fresh cilantro for garnish

Instructions:
1. Preheat oven to 375°F (190°C).
2. In a bowl, mix cooked quinoa, black beans, corn, salsa, cumin, salt, and pepper.
3. Stuff bell peppers with the quinoa mixture.
4. Bake for 25-30 minutes or until peppers are tender.
5. Garnish with fresh cilantro before serving.

19. Lemon Herb Grilled Tofu:
Ingredients:
- 1 block extra-firm tofu, pressed and sliced
- 2 tablespoons olive oil
- 2 tablespoons lemon juice
- 1 teaspoon dried thyme
- 1 teaspoon dried rosemary
- Salt and pepper to taste

Instructions:
1. Preheat grill to medium-high heat.
2. In a bowl, mix olive oil, lemon juice, dried thyme, dried rosemary, salt, and pepper.
3. Coat tofu slices with the marinade.
4. Grill tofu for 3-4 minutes per side or until grill marks appear.

20. Zucchini Noodles with Pesto Shrimp:
Ingredients:
- 1 pound shrimp, peeled and deveined
- 4 medium zucchini, spiralized into noodles
- 2 tablespoons olive oil
- 1/2 cup cherry tomatoes, halved
- 1/4 cup pesto sauce
- Salt and pepper to taste
- Parmesan cheese for garnish

Instructions:
1. In a skillet, heat olive oil over medium heat.

2. Add shrimp and cook until pink and opaque.

3. Stir in zucchini noodles and cherry tomatoes. Cook until noodles are tender.

4. Mix in pesto sauce and season with salt and pepper.

5. Garnish with Parmesan cheese before serving.

21. Mediterranean Quinoa Bowl:
Ingredients:
- 1 cup quinoa, cooked
- 1 cup cherry tomatoes, halved
- 1 cucumber, diced
- 1/4 cup Kalamata olives, sliced
- 1/4 cup feta cheese, crumbled
- 2 tablespoons olive oil
- 1 tablespoon red wine vinegar
- 1 teaspoon dried oregano
- Salt and pepper to taste

Instructions:
1. In a bowl, combine cooked quinoa, cherry tomatoes, cucumber, Kalamata olives, and feta cheese.
2. In a small bowl, whisk together olive oil, red wine vinegar, dried oregano, salt, and pepper.
3. Pour the dressing over the quinoa mixture and toss gently.
4. Serve as a refreshing and satisfying bowl.

22. Lentil and Vegetable Curry:
Ingredients:
- 1 cup dry lentils, rinsed and drained
- 1 tablespoon olive oil
- 1 onion, diced
- 2 cloves garlic, minced
- 1 tablespoon curry powder
- 1 can (14 oz) diced tomatoes
- 2 cups mixed vegetables (carrots, peas, bell peppers)
- 1 can (14 oz) coconut milk

- Salt and pepper to taste
- Fresh cilantro for garnish

Instructions:
1. Cook lentils according to package instructions.
2. In a skillet, heat olive oil over medium heat.
3. Add diced onions and cook until softened.
4. Add minced garlic and curry powder. Cook for 1 minute.
5. Stir in cooked lentils, diced tomatoes, mixed vegetables, and coconut milk.
6. Simmer until vegetables are tender.
7. Garnish with fresh cilantro before serving.

23. Cauliflower Fried Rice with Tofu:
Ingredients:
- 1 block extra-firm tofu, pressed and crumbled
- 1 head cauliflower, grated into rice-like consistency
- 2 tablespoons low-sodium soy sauce
- 1 tablespoon sesame oil
- 1 cup mixed vegetables (peas, carrots, corn)
- 2 cloves garlic, minced
- 1 tablespoon ginger, grated
- 2 green onions, sliced

Instructions:
1. In a wok or large skillet, sauté crumbled tofu until golden brown.
2. Add grated cauliflower, soy sauce, and sesame oil. Stir-fry until cauliflower is cooked.
3. Stir in mixed vegetables, minced garlic, grated ginger, and sliced green onions.
4. Cook until vegetables are tender.

24. Stuffed Cabbage Rolls:
Ingredients:
- 8 large cabbage leaves
- 1 cup quinoa, cooked
- 1 pound lean ground turkey

- 1 can (14 oz) diced tomatoes
- 1 teaspoon dried thyme
- 1 teaspoon smoked paprika
- Salt and pepper to taste
- Fresh parsley for garnish

Instructions:
1. Preheat oven to 375°F (190°C).
2. Blanch cabbage leaves in boiling water for 2-3 minutes. Drain and set aside.
3. In a bowl, mix cooked quinoa, ground turkey, diced tomatoes, dried thyme, smoked paprika, salt, and pepper.
4. Spoon the mixture onto each cabbage leaf and roll.
5. Place the rolls in a baking dish.
6. Bake for 25-30 minutes or until the rolls are heated through.
7. Garnish with fresh parsley before serving.

25. Moroccan Chickpea Stew:
Ingredients:
- 2 cans (15 oz each) chickpeas, drained and rinsed
- 1 tablespoon olive oil
- 1 onion, diced
- 2 cloves garlic, minced
- 1 teaspoon ground cumin
- 1 teaspoon ground coriander
- 1/2 teaspoon cinnamon
- 1 can (14 oz) diced tomatoes
- 4 cups vegetable broth
- 1 cup butternut squash, diced
- Salt and pepper to taste
- Fresh cilantro for garnish

Instructions:
1. In a large pot, sauté diced onions in olive oil until softened.
2. Add minced garlic, ground cumin, ground coriander, and cinnamon. Cook for 1 minute.

3. Stir in chickpeas, diced tomatoes, vegetable broth, diced butternut squash, salt, and pepper.
4. Simmer until butternut squash is tender.
5. Garnish with fresh cilantro before serving.

26. Shrimp and Quinoa Paella:
Ingredients:
- 1 pound shrimp, peeled and deveined
- 1 cup quinoa, cooked
- 1 onion, diced
- 2 bell peppers, diced
- 2 cloves garlic, minced
- 1 teaspoon smoked paprika
- 1/2 teaspoon saffron threads (optional)
- 1 can (14 oz) diced tomatoes
- 2 cups vegetable broth
- Fresh parsley for garnish

Instructions:
1. In a large skillet, sauté diced onions until softened.
2. Add diced bell peppers and minced garlic. Cook until vegetables are tender.
3. Stir in cooked quinoa, smoked paprika, saffron threads, diced tomatoes, and vegetable broth.
4. Arrange shrimp on top and cover. Cook until shrimp is pink and opaque.
5. Garnish with fresh parsley before serving.

27. Asian-Inspired Tofu and Vegetable Stir-Fry:
Ingredients:
- 1 block extra-firm tofu, pressed and cubed
- 2 tablespoons low-sodium soy sauce
- 1 tablespoon sesame oil
- 1 tablespoon rice vinegar
- 1 tablespoon honey
- 1 tablespoon olive oil
- Assorted vegetables (broccoli, bell peppers, snap peas)

Instructions:
1. In a bowl, mix soy sauce, sesame oil, rice vinegar, honey, and olive oil.
2. In a skillet, heat olive oil over medium heat.
3. Add cubed tofu and stir-fry until golden brown.
4. Add assorted vegetables and sauce mixture. Stir-fry until vegetables are tender.

28. Tomato Basil Turkey Meatballs:
Ingredients:
- 1 pound lean ground turkey
- 1/2 cup whole wheat breadcrumbs
- 1/4 cup grated Parmesan cheese
- 1 egg
- 2 cloves garlic, minced
- 1 teaspoon dried basil
- 1 can (14 oz) crushed tomatoes
- 1 teaspoon dried oregano
- Salt and pepper to taste
- Fresh basil for garnish

Instructions:
1. Preheat oven to 375°F (190°C).
2. In a bowl, combine ground turkey, breadcrumbs, Parmesan cheese, egg, minced garlic, and dried basil.
3. Shape the mixture into meatballs and place them on a baking sheet.
4. In a separate bowl, mix crushed tomatoes, dried oregano, salt, and pepper.
5. Spoon the tomato mixture over the meatballs.
6. Bake for 25-30 minutes or until meatballs are cooked through.
7. Garnish with fresh basil before serving.

29. Greek Lemon Chicken Skewers:
Ingredients:
- 1 pound boneless, skinless chicken breast, cut into cubes
- 1/4 cup olive oil
- 2 tablespoons lemon juice
- 2 cloves garlic, minced

- 1 teaspoon dried oregano
-Ingredients (Continued):
- 1 teaspoon dried thyme
- Salt and pepper to taste
- Cherry tomatoes
- Red onion, sliced

Instructions:
1. In a bowl, mix olive oil, lemon juice, minced garlic, dried oregano, dried thyme, salt, and pepper.
2. Coat chicken cubes with the marinade and let them marinate for at least 30 minutes.
3. Thread marinated chicken, cherry tomatoes, and sliced red onion onto skewers.
4. Grill skewers for 5-7 minutes per side or until chicken is cooked through.

30. Spinach and Feta Stuffed Chicken Breast:
Ingredients:
- 4 boneless, skinless chicken breasts
- 2 cups fresh spinach, chopped
- 1/2 cup feta cheese, crumbled
- 2 cloves garlic, minced
- 1 tablespoon olive oil
- 1 teaspoon dried oregano
- Salt and pepper to taste
- Lemon wedges for serving

Instructions:
1. Preheat oven to 400°F (200°C).
2. In a skillet, sauté chopped spinach, crumbled feta, minced garlic, olive oil, dried oregano, salt, and pepper until spinach is wilted.
3. Cut a pocket into each chicken breast.
4. Stuff each chicken breast with the spinach and feta mixture.
5. Secure the pockets with toothpicks if needed.
6. Place stuffed chicken breasts on a baking sheet and bake for 25-30 minutes or until chicken is cooked through.

7. Serve with lemon wedges for a burst of freshness.

Chapter 8: Side Dishes and Accompaniments

1. Roasted Brussels Sprouts:

Ingredients:

- Brussels sprouts, trimmed and halved
- Olive oil
- Garlic powder
- Salt and pepper to taste

Instructions:

1. Toss Brussels sprouts with olive oil, garlic powder, salt, and pepper.
2. Roast in the oven at 400°F (200°C) for 20-25 minutes or until crispy.

2. Quinoa Salad with Cucumber and Mint:

Ingredients:

- Cooked quinoa
- Cucumber, diced
- Fresh mint, chopped
- Olive oil
- Lemon juice
- Salt and pepper to taste

Instructions:

1. Combine cooked quinoa, diced cucumber, and chopped mint.
2. Drizzle with olive oil and lemon juice. Season with salt and pepper.

3. Steamed Asparagus with Lemon Butter:

Ingredients:

- Fresh asparagus, trimmed
- Butter
- Lemon zest
- Lemon juice
- Salt and pepper to taste

Instructions:
1. Steam asparagus until tender-crisp.
2. In a pan, melt butter and add lemon zest and juice.
3. Drizzle the lemon butter over the steamed asparagus. Season with salt and pepper.

4. Mashed Sweet Potatoes:
Ingredients:
- Sweet potatoes, peeled and diced
- Olive oil
- Nutmeg
- Salt and pepper to taste

Instructions:
1. Boil or steam sweet potatoes until tender.
2. Mash with olive oil, a pinch of nutmeg, salt, and pepper.

5. Lemon Herb Quinoa:
Ingredients:
- Cooked quinoa
- Lemon zest
- Fresh herbs (parsley, dill, chives), chopped
- Olive oil
- Salt and pepper to taste

Instructions:
1. Mix cooked quinoa with lemon zest, fresh herbs, and olive oil.
2. Season with salt and pepper.

6. Baked Sweet Potato Fries:
Ingredients:
- Sweet potatoes, cut into fries
- Olive oil
- Paprika
- Garlic powder

- Salt and pepper to taste

Instructions:
1. Toss sweet potato fries with olive oil, paprika, garlic powder, salt, and pepper.
2. Bake in the oven at 425°F (220°C) for 20-25 minutes or until crispy.

7. Sauteed Spinach with Garlic:
Ingredients:
- Fresh spinach
- Olive oil
- Garlic, minced
- Lemon juice
- Salt and pepper to taste

Instructions:
1. In a pan, sauté minced garlic in olive oil until fragrant.
2. Add fresh spinach and sauté until wilted.
3. Drizzle with lemon juice and season with salt and pepper.

8. Cauliflower Mash:
Ingredients:
- Cauliflower florets
- Chicken or vegetable broth
- Olive oil
- Garlic powder
- Salt and pepper to taste

Instructions:
1. Steam cauliflower until very tender.
2. Mash with broth, olive oil, garlic powder, salt, and pepper.

9. Caprese Salad:
Ingredients:
- Tomatoes, sliced
- Fresh mozzarella, sliced

- Fresh basil leaves
- Balsamic glaze
- Olive oil
- Salt and pepper to taste

Instructions:
1. Arrange tomato and mozzarella slices on a plate.
2. Top with fresh basil leaves.
3. Drizzle with balsamic glaze and olive oil. Season with salt and pepper.

10. Grilled Zucchini with Herbs:
Ingredients:
- Zucchini, sliced
- Olive oil
- Fresh herbs (rosemary, thyme), chopped
- Lemon zest
- Salt and pepper to taste

Instructions:
1. Brush zucchini slices with olive oil.
2. Grill until tender. Sprinkle with fresh herbs, lemon zest, salt, and pepper.

11. Brown Rice Pilaf:
Ingredients:
- Cooked brown rice
- Slivered almonds
- Dried cranberries
- Fresh parsley, chopped
- Olive oil
- Salt and pepper to taste

Instructions:
1. Combine brown rice with slivered almonds, dried cranberries, and chopped parsley.
2. Drizzle with olive oil. Season with salt and pepper.

12. Cucumber Avocado Salad:
Ingredients:
- Cucumber, diced
- Avocado, diced
- Red onion, finely chopped
- Fresh cilantro, chopped
- Lime juice
- Salt and pepper to taste

Instructions:
1. Mix cucumber, avocado, red onion, and cilantro.
2. Drizzle with lime juice. Season with salt and pepper.

13. Baked Parmesan Zucchini Rounds:
Ingredients:
- Zucchini, sliced
- Parmesan cheese, grated
- Olive oil
- Garlic powder
- Salt and pepper to taste

Instructions:
1. Arrange zucchini slices on a baking sheet.
2. Drizzle with olive oil and sprinkle with Parmesan, garlic powder, salt, and pepper.
3. Bake at 400°F (200°C) for 15-20 minutes or until golden.

14. Mediterranean Chickpea Salad:
Ingredients:
- Canned chickpeas, drained and rinsed
- Cherry tomatoes, halved
- Cucumber, diced
- Red onion, finely chopped
- Kalamata olives, sliced
- Feta cheese, crumbled

- Olive oil
- Lemon juice
- Fresh oregano, chopped
- Salt and pepper to taste

Instructions:
1. Combine chickpeas, cherry tomatoes, cucumber, red onion, Kalamata olives, and feta cheese.
2. Drizzle with olive oil and lemon juice. Sprinkle with fresh oregano. Season with salt and pepper.

15. Herb-Roasted Carrots:
Ingredients:
- Carrots, peeled and cut into sticks
- Olive oil
- Fresh herbs (thyme, rosemary), chopped
- Honey (optional)
- Salt and pepper to taste

Instructions:
1. Toss carrot sticks with olive oil, fresh herbs, honey (optional), salt, and pepper.
2. Roast in the oven at 400°F (200°C) for 20-25 minutes or until caramelized.

16. Ratatouille:
Ingredients:
- Eggplant, diced
- Zucchini, sliced
- Bell peppers, diced
- Onion, diced
- Garlic, minced
- Tomatoes, diced
- Fresh basil, chopped
- Olive oil
- Herbes de Provence
- Salt and pepper to taste

Instructions:
1. Sauté onions and garlic in olive oil until softened.
2. Add diced eggplant, sliced zucchini, diced bell peppers, and tomatoes.
3. Season with fresh basil, Herbes de Provence, salt, and pepper. Simmer until vegetables are tender.

17. Lemon Garlic Green Beans:
Ingredients:
- Fresh green beans, trimmed
- Olive oil
- Lemon zest
- Garlic, minced
- Almonds, sliced
- Salt and pepper to taste

Instructions:
1. Steam green beans until crisp-tender.
2. Sauté minced garlic in olive oil until fragrant.
3. Toss green beans with garlic oil, lemon zest, sliced almonds, salt, and pepper.

18. Spinach and Mushroom Saute:
Ingredients:
- Fresh spinach
- Mushrooms, sliced
- Olive oil
- Garlic, minced
- Lemon juice
- Salt and pepper to taste

Instructions:
1. Sauté mushrooms and minced garlic in olive oil until mushrooms are golden.
2. Add fresh spinach and sauté until wilted.
3. Drizzle with lemon juice. Season with salt and pepper.

19. Balsamic Glazed Roasted Vegetables:
Ingredients:
- Assorted vegetables (carrots, bell peppers, onions, cherry tomatoes)
- Olive oil
- Balsamic glaze
- Fresh thyme, chopped
- Salt and pepper to taste

Instructions:
1. Toss assorted vegetables with olive oil, balsamic glaze, fresh thyme, salt, and pepper.
2. Roast in the oven at 425°F (220°C) for 20-25 minutes or until caramelized.

20. Greek Tzatziki Sauce:
Ingredients:
- Greek yogurt
- Cucumber, grated and drained
- Garlic, minced
- Fresh dill, chopped
- Lemon juice
- Salt and pepper to taste

Instructions:
1. Mix Greek yogurt with grated cucumber, minced garlic, fresh dill, lemon juice, salt, and pepper.
2. Chill before serving. Use as a refreshing dip or sauce.

Chapter 9: Sweet Treats

1. Baked Apples with Cinnamon:
Ingredients:
- Apples, cored and sliced
- Cinnamon
- Nutmeg
- Honey (optional)

Instructions:
1. Place apple slices in a baking dish.
2. Sprinkle with cinnamon and nutmeg.
3. Drizzle with honey if desired.
4. Bake at 350°F (175°C) for 20-25 minutes or until tender.

2. Berry Parfait:
Ingredients:
- Mixed berries (strawberries, blueberries, raspberries)
- Greek yogurt
- Granola (low-fat)

Instructions:
1. Layer Greek yogurt, mixed berries, and granola in a glass.
2. Repeat the layers.
3. Top with a dollop of Greek yogurt and a few berries.

3. Banana-Oat Cookies:
Ingredients:
- Ripe bananas, mashed
- Rolled oats
- Cinnamon
- Vanilla extract
- Nuts or seeds (optional)

Instructions:
1. Mix mashed bananas, rolled oats, cinnamon, vanilla extract, and nuts/seeds.
2. Drop spoonfuls onto a baking sheet.
3. Bake at 350°F (175°C) for 15-20 minutes or until golden.

4. Chia Seed Pudding:
Ingredients:
- Chia seeds
- Almond milk
- Vanilla extract
- Maple syrup (optional)
- Fresh fruit for topping

Instructions:
1. Mix chia seeds, almond milk, vanilla extract, and maple syrup in a jar.
2. Refrigerate for at least 4 hours or overnight.
3. Top with fresh fruit before serving.

5. Mango Sorbet:
Ingredients:
- Ripe mangoes, peeled and diced
- Lime juice
- Honey (optional)

Instructions:
1. Blend diced mangoes, lime juice, and honey (if using) until smooth.
2. Pour into a shallow dish and freeze.
3. Scoop out with an ice cream scoop when ready to serve.

6. Dark Chocolate-Dipped Strawberries:
Ingredients:
- Fresh strawberries, washed and dried
- Dark chocolate (70% cocoa or higher)

Instructions:

1. Melt dark chocolate in a heatproof bowl.

2. Dip each strawberry into the melted chocolate.

3. Place on parchment paper and let it set.

7. Cinnamon Roasted Almonds:

Ingredients:

- Raw almonds

- Cinnamon

- Honey (optional)

Instructions:

1. Toss raw almonds with cinnamon.

2. Roast in the oven at 325°F (160°C) for 10-15 minutes.

3. Drizzle with honey if desired.

8. Poached Pears with Vanilla Yogurt:

Ingredients:

- Pears, peeled and halved

- Water

- Vanilla extract

- Greek yogurt

Instructions:

1. Poach pears in water with a splash of vanilla extract until tender.

2. Serve with a dollop of Greek yogurt.

9. Baked Peach with Cinnamon and Yogurt:

Ingredients:

- Ripe peaches, halved and pitted

- Cinnamon

- Greek yogurt

Instructions:

1. Place peach halves in a baking dish.

2. Sprinkle with cinnamon.
3. Bake at 375°F (190°C) for 20-25 minutes.
4. Serve with a spoonful of Greek yogurt.

10. Coconut and Lime Energy Balls:
Ingredients:
- Dates, pitted
- Shredded coconut
- Lime zest
- Almond meal

Instructions:
1. Blend dates, shredded coconut, lime zest, and almond meal in a food processor.
2. Roll into small balls and refrigerate.

11. Vanilla Chia Seed Pudding with Fresh Berries:
Ingredients:
- Chia seeds
- Almond milk
- Vanilla extract
- Maple syrup (optional)
- Mixed berries for topping

Instructions:
1. Mix chia seeds, almond milk, vanilla extract, and maple syrup in a jar.
2. Refrigerate for at least 4 hours or overnight.
3. Top with fresh mixed berries before serving.

12. Frozen Banana Bites:
Ingredients:
- Ripe bananas, sliced
- Almond butter
- Dark chocolate (70% cocoa or higher), melted

Instructions:
1. Spread almond butter on banana slices.
2. Sandwich them together and freeze.
3. Dip the frozen banana bites in melted dark chocolate.

13. Baked Cinnamon-Pecan Apples:
Ingredients:
- Apples, cored and sliced
- Cinnamon
- Chopped pecans
- Maple syrup (optional)

Instructions:
1. Place apple slices in a baking dish.
2. Sprinkle with cinnamon and chopped pecans.
3. Drizzle with maple syrup if desired.
4. Bake at 350°F (175°C) for 20-25 minutes or until tender.

14. Coconut Lime Sorbet:
Ingredients:
- Coconut milk
- Lime juice
- Shredded coconut (unsweetened)
- Agave syrup (optional)

Instructions:
1. Blend coconut milk, lime juice, shredded coconut, and agave syrup (if using) until smooth.
2. Pour into a shallow dish and freeze.
3. Scoop out with an ice cream scoop when ready to serve.

15. Cacao-Dusted Almond Dates:
Ingredients:
- Medjool dates, pitted
- Raw almonds

- Cacao powder

Instructions:
1. Stuff each date with a raw almond.
2. Roll in cacao powder until coated.

16. Peach and Raspberry Yogurt Parfait:
Ingredients:
- Fresh peaches, diced
- Raspberries
- Greek yogurt
- Honey (optional)

Instructions:
1. Layer diced peaches, raspberries, and Greek yogurt in a glass.
2. Repeat the layers.
3. Drizzle with honey if desired.

17. Pistachio and Fig Energy Bites:
Ingredients:
- Dried figs, stemmed
- Pistachios
- Rolled oats
- Honey
- Vanilla extract

Instructions:
1. Blend dried figs, pistachios, rolled oats, honey, and vanilla extract in a food processor.
2. Roll into small energy bites.

18. Baked Pears with Cinnamon and Walnuts:
Ingredients:
- Pears, halved and cored
- Cinnamon

- Chopped walnuts
- Maple syrup (optional)

Instructions:
1. Place pear halves in a baking dish.
2. Sprinkle with cinnamon and chopped walnuts.
3. Drizzle with maple syrup if desired.
4. Bake at 375°F (190°C) for 20-25 minutes.

19. Blueberry and Lemon Frozen Yogurt Bites:
Ingredients:
- Greek yogurt
- Fresh blueberries
- Lemon zest
- Maple syrup (optional)

Instructions:
1. Mix Greek yogurt, fresh blueberries, lemon zest, and maple syrup (if using).
2. Spoon into small molds or ice cube trays.
3. Freeze until solid.

20. Date and Walnut Bliss Balls:
Ingredients:
- Dates, pitted
- Walnuts
- Shredded coconut (unsweetened)

Instructions:
1. Blend dates and walnuts in a food processor until a sticky dough forms.
2. Roll into small bliss balls and coat with shredded coconut.

Chapter 10: 4 Weeks Meal Plan and Batch Cooking

A. Weekly Meal Planning Tips + 4 weeks meal plan to reverse pancreatitis

Weekly Meal Planning Tips for Pancreatitis:

1. Focus on Low-Fat Options:
   - Choose lean protein sources such as poultry, fish, tofu, and legumes.
   - Opt for low-fat or fat-free dairy products.
   - Limit or avoid fried and fatty foods.

2. Include Whole Grains:
   - Embrace whole grains like brown rice, quinoa, and whole wheat.
   - These provide essential nutrients and fiber without excessive fat.

3. Load Up on Fruits and Vegetables:
   - Incorporate a variety of colorful fruits and vegetables.
   - Opt for cooked or steamed vegetables to ease digestion.

4. Choose Low-Fat Cooking Methods:
   - Use cooking methods like baking, grilling, steaming, and sautéing with minimal oil.
   - Avoid heavy sauces and gravies.

5. Stay Hydrated:
   - Drink plenty of water throughout the day to stay hydrated.
   - Limit or avoid sugary beverages and caffeinated drinks.

6. Manage Portion Sizes:
   - Pay attention to portion sizes to prevent overeating.
   - Eating smaller, frequent meals may be easier on the digestive system.

7. Limit Processed and High-Sugar Foods:

- Minimize processed foods and those high in added sugars.
- Opt for natural sweetness from fruits.

8. Be Mindful of Trigger Foods:
   - Identify and avoid foods that trigger discomfort or exacerbate symptoms.
   - Keep a food diary to track reactions.

9. Incorporate Healthy Fats:
   - Include sources of healthy fats like avocados, nuts, and olive oil in moderation.
   - These can provide essential nutrients without overloading the pancreas.

10. Plan Balanced Meals:
   - Aim for a balance of carbohydrates, proteins, and fats in each meal.
   - Include a variety of nutrient-dense foods.

4-Week Meal Plan to Reverse Pancreatitis:

Week 1:

Day 1:
- **Breakfast:**
  - **Oatmeal with sliced banana, a sprinkle of cinnamon, and a dollop of Greek yogurt.**
- **Lunch:**
  - **Grilled chicken breast with quinoa and steamed broccoli.**
- **Dinner:**
  - **Baked salmon with sweet potato wedges and sautéed spinach.**

Day 2:
- **Breakfast:**
  - **Whole-grain toast with avocado slices and poached eggs.**
- **Lunch:**
  - **Lentil soup with a side of mixed greens salad.**
- **Dinner:**
  - **Stir-fried tofu with brown rice and a medley of colorful vegetables.**

Day 3:
- Breakfast:
  - Greek yogurt parfait with fresh berries, chia seeds, and a drizzle of honey.
- Lunch:
  - Turkey and vegetable wrap with whole-grain tortilla and a side of carrot sticks.
- Dinner:
  - Quinoa salad with cucumber, cherry tomatoes, feta cheese, and lemon vinaigrette.

Day 4:
- Breakfast:
  - Smoothie with spinach, banana, almond milk, and a scoop of protein powder.
- Lunch:
  - Baked cod with quinoa and roasted Brussels sprouts.
- Dinner:
  - Chickpea and vegetable curry with brown rice.

Day 5:
- Breakfast:
  - Whole-grain pancakes with fresh berries and a drizzle of pure maple syrup.
- Lunch:
  - Grilled shrimp salad with mixed greens, cherry tomatoes, and balsamic vinaigrette.
- Dinner:
  - Baked chicken breast with wild rice and steamed asparagus.

Day 6:
- Breakfast:
  - Overnight chia seed pudding with almond milk, topped with sliced strawberries.
- Lunch:
  - Quinoa bowl with black beans, corn, avocado, and a squeeze of lime.

- Dinner:
  - Grilled vegetable skewers with a side of couscous.

Day 7:
- Breakfast:
  - Whole-grain waffles with Greek yogurt and mixed fruit compote.
- Lunch:
  - Lentil and vegetable stir-fry with brown rice.
- Dinner:
  - Turkey meatballs with whole-grain spaghetti and tomato sauce.

Week 2:

Day 8:
- Breakfast:
  - Smoothie with kale, pineapple, banana, and almond milk.
- Lunch:
  - Grilled chicken salad with mixed greens, cherry tomatoes, and a light vinaigrette.
- Dinner:
  - Baked trout with quinoa pilaf and steamed asparagus.

Day 9:
- Breakfast:
  - Greek yogurt with sliced peaches and a sprinkle of chopped almonds.
- Lunch:
  - Lentil and vegetable wrap with whole-grain tortilla and a side of cucumber slices.
- Dinner:
  - Stir-fried tofu with broccoli and brown rice.

Day 10:
- Breakfast:
  - Whole-grain toast with avocado and smoked salmon.
- Lunch:

- Chickpea and vegetable curry with quinoa.
- Dinner:
  - Baked chicken breast with sweet potato mash and sautéed green beans.

Day 11:
- Breakfast:
  - Overnight chia seed pudding with almond milk, topped with mixed berries.
- Lunch:
  - Turkey and vegetable stir-fry with brown rice.
- Dinner:
  - Grilled shrimp with quinoa and roasted Brussels sprouts.

Day 12:
- Breakfast:
  - Whole-grain pancakes with fresh strawberries and a drizzle of honey.
- Lunch:
  - Quinoa salad with cucumber, cherry tomatoes, feta cheese, and lemon vinaigrette.
- Dinner:
  - Baked cod with quinoa and sautéed spinach.

Day 13:
- Breakfast:
  - Oatmeal with sliced banana, a sprinkle of cinnamon, and a dollop of Greek yogurt.
- Lunch:
  - Lentil soup with a side of mixed greens salad.
- Dinner:
  - Stir-fried tofu with brown rice and a medley of colorful vegetables.

Day 14:
- Breakfast:
  - Greek yogurt parfait with fresh berries, chia seeds, and a drizzle of honey.
- Lunch:

- Turkey and vegetable wrap with whole-grain tortilla and a side of carrot sticks.
- Dinner:
 - Quinoa salad with cucumber, cherry tomatoes, feta cheese, and lemon vinaigrette.
 Week 3:

 Day 15:
- Breakfast:
 - Smoothie with spinach, mango, banana, and almond milk.
- Lunch:
 - Grilled chicken salad with mixed greens, cherry tomatoes, and a light balsamic vinaigrette.
- Dinner:
 - Baked salmon with quinoa and roasted Brussels sprouts.

 Day 16:
- Breakfast:
 - Greek yogurt with sliced peaches and a sprinkle of chopped almonds.
- Lunch:
 - Lentil and vegetable stir-fry with brown rice.
- Dinner:
 - Stir-fried tofu with broccoli and quinoa.

 Day 17:
- Breakfast:
 - Whole-grain toast with avocado and smoked salmon.
- Lunch:
 - Chickpea and vegetable curry with quinoa.
- Dinner:
 - Baked chicken breast with sweet potato mash and steamed asparagus.

 Day 18:
- Breakfast:
 - Overnight chia seed pudding with almond milk, topped with mixed berries.

- Lunch:
  - Turkey and vegetable wrap with whole-grain tortilla and a side of cucumber slices.
- Dinner:
  - Grilled shrimp with quinoa and sautéed green beans.
 Day 19:
- Breakfast:
  - Whole-grain pancakes with fresh strawberries and a drizzle of honey.
- Lunch:
  - Quinoa salad with cucumber, cherry tomatoes, feta cheese, and lemon vinaigrette.
- Dinner:
  - Baked cod with quinoa and steamed broccoli.

 Day 20:
- Breakfast:
  - Oatmeal with sliced banana, a sprinkle of cinnamon, and a dollop of Greek yogurt.
- Lunch:
  - Lentil soup with a side of mixed greens salad.
- Dinner:
  - Stir-fried tofu with brown rice and a medley of colorful vegetables.

 Day 21:
- Breakfast:
  - Greek yogurt parfait with fresh berries, chia seeds, and a drizzle of honey.
- Lunch:
  - Turkey and vegetable wrap with whole-grain tortilla and a side of carrot sticks.
- Dinner:
  - Quinoa salad with cucumber, cherry tomatoes, feta cheese, and lemon vinaigrette.

 Week 4:

Day 22:
- Breakfast:
 - Smoothie with kale, pineapple, banana, and almond milk.
- Lunch:
 - Grilled chicken salad with mixed greens, cherry tomatoes, and a light balsamic vinaigrette.
- Dinner:
 - Baked salmon with quinoa and roasted Brussels sprouts.

Day 23:
- Breakfast:
 - Greek yogurt with sliced peaches and a sprinkle of chopped almonds.
- Lunch:
 - Lentil and vegetable stir-fry with brown rice.
- Dinner:
 - Stir-fried tofu with broccoli and quinoa.

Day 24:
- Breakfast:
 - Whole-grain toast with avocado and smoked salmon.
- Lunch:
 - Chickpea and vegetable curry with quinoa.
- Dinner:
 - Baked chicken breast with sweet potato mash and steamed asparagus.

Day 25:
- Breakfast:
 - Overnight chia seed pudding with almond milk, topped with mixed berries.
- Lunch:
 - Turkey and vegetable wrap with whole-grain tortilla and a side of cucumber slices.
- Dinner:
 - Grilled shrimp with quinoa and sautéed green beans.

Day 26:

- Breakfast:
 - Whole-grain pancakes with fresh strawberries and a drizzle of honey.
- Lunch:
  - Quinoa salad with cucumber, cherry tomatoes, feta cheese, and lemon vinaigrette.

- Dinner:
 - Baked cod with quinoa and steamed broccoli.

Day 27:
- Breakfast:
 - Oatmeal with sliced banana, a sprinkle of cinnamon, and a dollop of Greek yogurt.
- Lunch:
 - Lentil soup with a side of mixed greens salad.
- Dinner:
 - Stir-fried tofu with brown rice and a medley of colorful vegetables.

Day 28:
- Breakfast:
 - Greek yogurt parfait with fresh berries, chia seeds, and a drizzle of honey.
- Lunch:
 - Turkey and vegetable wrap with whole-grain tortilla and a side of carrot sticks.
- Dinner:
  - Quinoa salad with cucumber, cherry tomatoes, feta cheese, and lemon vinaigrette.

B. Batch Cooking Strategies

Batch cooking is a great strategy to save time, simplify meal preparation, and ensure that you have wholesome meals readily available, especially when following a specific dietary plan like one for pancreatitis. Here are some batch cooking strategies to help you efficiently plan and prepare your meals:

1. Meal Planning:

- Create a Weekly Menu: Plan your meals for the week, including breakfast, lunch, dinner, and snacks. This will guide your batch cooking efforts.
- Variety: Ensure a variety of proteins, grains, vegetables, and fruits to meet your nutritional needs.

2. Batch Cooking Basics:
- Select Versatile Ingredients: Choose ingredients that can be used in multiple dishes. For example, if you cook a batch of grilled chicken, you can use it in salads, wraps, or stir-fries.
- Cook in Batches: Prepare larger quantities of staple items like grains (quinoa, rice), proteins, and vegetables at once.

3. Storage and Portioning:
- Invest in Quality Containers: Use airtight containers to store cooked food. Consider portion-sized containers for easy grab-and-go meals.
- Labeling: Clearly label containers with the date of preparation to monitor freshness.
- Freezing: Freeze portions of meals that may not be consumed within a few days.

4. Cooking Sessions:
- Dedicated Batch Cooking Day: Set aside a specific day in the week for batch cooking. This can be a time-saving and stress-free approach.
- Efficient Workflow: Plan your cooking sessions with an efficient workflow to minimize time in the kitchen. For example, while one dish is simmering, you can prep ingredients for another.

5. Batch Cooking Ideas for Pancreatitis:
- Cook Proteins in Bulk: Grill or bake lean proteins such as chicken, turkey, or fish. Portion them into smaller servings.
- Prepare Grains and Legumes: Cook larger batches of whole grains (quinoa, brown rice) and legumes (lentils, chickpeas).

- Chop and Freeze Vegetables: Chop vegetables and freeze them for use in stir-fries, soups, or omelets.

- Soups and Stews: Prepare nutrient-dense soups and stews in larger quantities. Freeze individual servings for later use.

6. Adapt Recipes for Batch Cooking:

- Scale Recipes: Adjust recipe quantities to yield more servings. Use tools or apps to calculate ingredient amounts.

- One-Pot or Sheet Pan Meals: Opt for recipes that can be cooked in one pot or on a single sheet pan for easier cleanup.

7. Stay Organized:

- Inventory Tracking: Keep track of the items in your freezer and pantry to avoid food waste.

- Meal Rotation: Plan your meals to use older batches first, ensuring freshness.

8. Safety Considerations:

- Cooling Before Storage: Allow cooked items to cool before storing them in the refrigerator or freezer to prevent bacterial growth.

- Thawing: Follow safe thawing practices, especially when using frozen batches.

By incorporating these batch cooking strategies into your routine, you can make the process of meal preparation more efficient and support your pancreatitis-friendly diet with wholesome and readily available options.

C. Freezing and Storing Pancreatitis-Friendly Meals

Freezing and storing pancreatitis-friendly meals require careful attention to maintain the quality and safety of the food. Here are some guidelines to help you freeze and store your meals effectively:

1. Choose Suitable Containers:

- Airtight Containers: Use containers that provide an airtight seal to prevent freezer burn and maintain freshness.

- Freezer Bags: Consider using quality freezer bags for liquids or items with a higher moisture content.

2. Portion Control:
   - Single Servings: Portion your meals into single servings to avoid thawing more than needed.
   - Labeling: Clearly label each container with the name of the dish and the date of preparation.

3. Preparation Techniques:
   - Fully Cooked: Cook meals thoroughly before freezing. This ensures that the reheating process is minimal and safe.
   - Cooling: Allow cooked meals to cool completely before freezing to prevent condensation and ice crystals.

4. Freezing Techniques:
   - Flash Freezing: For items like vegetables, berries, or individual portions, spread them out on a baking sheet to freeze individually before transferring to containers.
   - Liquid Items: Leave some headspace in containers for liquids to expand as they freeze.

5. Pancreatitis-Friendly Meal Ideas for Freezing:
   - Lean Proteins: Freeze grilled chicken, turkey meatballs, or baked fish fillets.
   - Whole Grains: Portion cooked quinoa, brown rice, or other whole grains into containers.
   - Soups and Stews: Prepare nutrient-dense soups and stews and freeze them in individual servings.
   - Vegetables: Freeze chopped vegetables for use in stir-fries, omelets, or side dishes.
   - Sauces: Portion out pancreatitis-friendly sauces such as tomato sauce or vegetable-based sauces.

6. Thawing and Reheating:
   - Refrigerator Thawing: Thaw frozen meals in the refrigerator to maintain food safety.

- Microwave Reheating: Reheat meals in the microwave using microwave-safe containers.
- Stovetop or Oven: For larger items or meals, consider reheating on the stovetop or in the oven for even heating.

7. Storage Duration:
- Label with Dates: Clearly label each container with the date of preparation and use a "first in, first out" system.
- Storage Duration: Most frozen meals maintain quality for 1-3 months. Be mindful of the recommended storage duration for each type of meal.

8. Safety Considerations:
- Avoid Repeated Thawing and Freezing: Once thawed, avoid refreezing meals to maintain quality and safety.
- Check for Signs of Spoilage: Inspect frozen meals for any signs of freezer burn, off odors, or changes in texture.

9. Meal Rotation:
- Regular Inventory Check: Periodically check your freezer inventory to ensure that older items are used first.

10. Specific Considerations for Pancreatitis:
- Low-Fat Content: Ensure that the frozen meals adhere to your low-fat dietary requirements.
- Avoid High-Fat Sauces: Limit the use of high-fat sauces or gravies, as they may separate upon thawing and reheating.

Chapter 11: Dining Out with Pancreatitis

Dining out with pancreatitis can present challenges, but with careful consideration and communication, you can enjoy social gatherings without compromising your health. Here's a guide to making smart menu choices, communicating dietary needs to restaurants, and enjoying dining experiences while managing pancreatitis:

A. Making Smart Menu Choices:

1. Opt for Grilled or Baked Proteins:
   - Choose lean protein options such as grilled chicken, turkey, or fish.
   - Avoid fried or heavily sauced dishes that may be high in fat.

2. Choose Whole Grains:
   - Opt for dishes with whole grains like brown rice, quinoa, or whole wheat bread.
   - Avoid fried or buttered grains and opt for simple preparations.

3. Embrace Vegetables:
   - Select vegetable-based dishes, salads, and side dishes.
   - Request vegetables to be steamed or lightly sautéed without excessive oil.

4. Limit High-Fat Additions:
   - Be cautious with high-fat condiments, dressings, and sauces.
   - Ask for sauces on the side to control the amount you consume.

5. Mindful Beverage Choices:
   - Choose water, herbal teas, or diluted fruit juices instead of sugary or caffeinated drinks.
   - Limit alcohol consumption, as it can be irritating to the pancreas.

6. Control Portion Sizes:
   - Consider ordering appetizers or half portions to control the quantity of food.
   - Be mindful of portion sizes to avoid overeating.

B. Communicating Dietary Needs to Restaurants:

1. Inform Your Server:
   - Clearly communicate your dietary restrictions and preferences to your server.
   - Mention that you are managing pancreatitis and need to follow a low-fat dict.

2. Ask Questions:
   - Inquire about specific ingredients, cooking methods, and potential substitutions.
   - Request modifications to suit your dietary requirements.

3. Request Customizations:
   - Don't hesitate to ask for modifications to menu items to make them pancreatitis-friendly.
   - Ask for dishes to be prepared with minimal oil or without high-fat components.

4. Use Keywords:
   - Mention specific keywords related to your dietary needs, such as "low-fat," "grilled," or "steamed."
   - Restaurants are often familiar with these terms and can better accommodate your requests.

C. Enjoying Social Gatherings Without Compromising Health:

1. Plan Ahead:
   - Check the restaurant's menu online before going to have an idea of available options.
   - Choose restaurants with a variety of healthy choices.

2. Eat Mindfully:
   - Pay attention to hunger and fullness cues.
   - Take your time to enjoy each bite, and stop eating when satisfied.

3. Be Prepared to Educate:
   - Understand that not all restaurant staff may be familiar with pancreatitis.
   - Be prepared to provide brief explanations if necessary.

4. Bring Snacks:
   - Have a small, pancreatitis-friendly snack before going out to curb excessive hunger.
   - Carry a small snack with you in case of limited options.

5. Choose Restaurants Wisely:
   - Select restaurants with a reputation for accommodating dietary needs.
   - Ethnic restaurants often offer healthier options like grilled meats and fresh vegetables.

Remember to prioritize your health, and don't hesitate to advocate for your dietary needs when dining out. By making informed choices and communicating effectively, you can enjoy social gatherings while managing pancreatitis.

Chapter 12:   Wellness Beyond the Plate: Nurturing Holistic Health in Pancreatitis Management

Pancreatitis management extends beyond dietary considerations, embracing a holistic approach that prioritizes overall well-being. Incorporating stress management techniques, engaging in purposeful physical activity, cultivating a robust support system, and vigilantly monitoring progress form the cornerstones of a comprehensive wellness plan.

 A. Stress Management Techniques:

1. Mindfulness Meditation:
   - Embark on a journey of mindfulness through meditation. Devote time to practices like deep breathing, body scan, or guided meditation.
   - Cultivate awareness of your thoughts and sensations, fostering a sense of calm amid life's complexities.

2. Yoga and Stretching:
   - Integrate the therapeutic benefits of yoga into your routine. Gentle poses and stretches not only enhance physical flexibility but also contribute to mental relaxation.
   - Yoga encourages the union of mind and body, providing a holistic approach to stress reduction.

3. Journaling:
   - Establish a reflective practice through journaling. Record thoughts, emotions, and daily experiences.
   - Journaling serves as a valuable tool for self-discovery, helping you identify stress triggers and patterns.

4. Nature Walks:
   - Immerse yourself in the healing embrace of nature. Whether it's a serene walk in the park or an invigorating hike, time spent outdoors can alleviate stress.

- Nature's tranquility has a profound impact on mental well-being, offering a respite from the demands of daily life.

B. Physical Activity Recommendations:

1. Low-Impact Exercises:
- Prioritize low-impact exercises tailored to your fitness level. Activities like walking, swimming, or cycling foster cardiovascular health without undue strain.
- Regular, gentle movement contributes to overall vitality and supports the body's healing process.

2. Strength Training:
- Introduce strength training into your routine using light weights or resistance bands. This promotes muscle strength and endurance.
- A personalized strength training program, approved by healthcare professionals, can enhance physical resilience.

3. Consult with a Professional:
- Seek guidance from healthcare professionals before initiating any exercise regimen. They can provide insights into safe and effective activities based on your health condition.
- Regular check-ins with healthcare providers ensure that your physical activity aligns with your unique health requirements.

C. Building a Support System:

1. Connect with Others:
- Forge connections with individuals sharing similar health challenges. Join support groups, either locally or online, to exchange experiences and insights.
- Shared experiences foster a sense of understanding and camaraderie.

2. Involve Loved Ones:
- Foster open communication with friends and family about your health journey. Educate them about pancreatitis and your specific dietary needs.

- Involving loved ones creates a supportive environment that contributes to emotional well-being.

3. Support Groups:
  - Actively participate in support groups designed for those managing pancrcatitis. Engage in discussions, share coping strategies, and learn from the collective wisdom of the community.
  - Online forums and local support groups offer a platform for mutual encouragement.

D. Monitoring Progress and Adjusting as Needed:

1. Regular Health Check-ups:
  - Schedule regular check-ups with healthcare providers to monitor pancreatitis indicators. These evaluations guide adjustments to your wellness plan.
  - Routine check-ups ensure that your overall health is monitored, enabling early intervention if needed.

2. Keep a Wellness Journal:
  - Maintain a comprehensive wellness journal to track dietary choices, physical activity, stress levels, and emotional well-being.
  - The journal serves as a dynamic tool for self-reflection, aiding in the identification of patterns and triggers.

3. Adjusting Lifestyle:
  - Embrace flexibility in adapting lifestyle choices. If certain activities or foods no longer support your well-being, be open to making thoughtful adjustments.
  - Periodically reassess your wellness plan to align it with evolving health needs.

4. Celebrate Achievements:
  - Acknowledge and celebrate milestones achieved on your wellness journey, irrespective of their scale. Recognizing progress, no matter how modest, fosters a positive mindset.
  - Small victories contribute to sustained motivation and resilience.

In cultivating a holistic wellness plan, remember that individual needs vary. Collaborate closely with healthcare professionals to tailor your plan to your unique circumstances. A harmonious integration of stress management, purposeful physical activity, a strong support system, and vigilant progress monitoring lays the foundation for a robust and resilient well-being in the face of pancreatitis management.